The Diabetic's Sports and Exercise Book

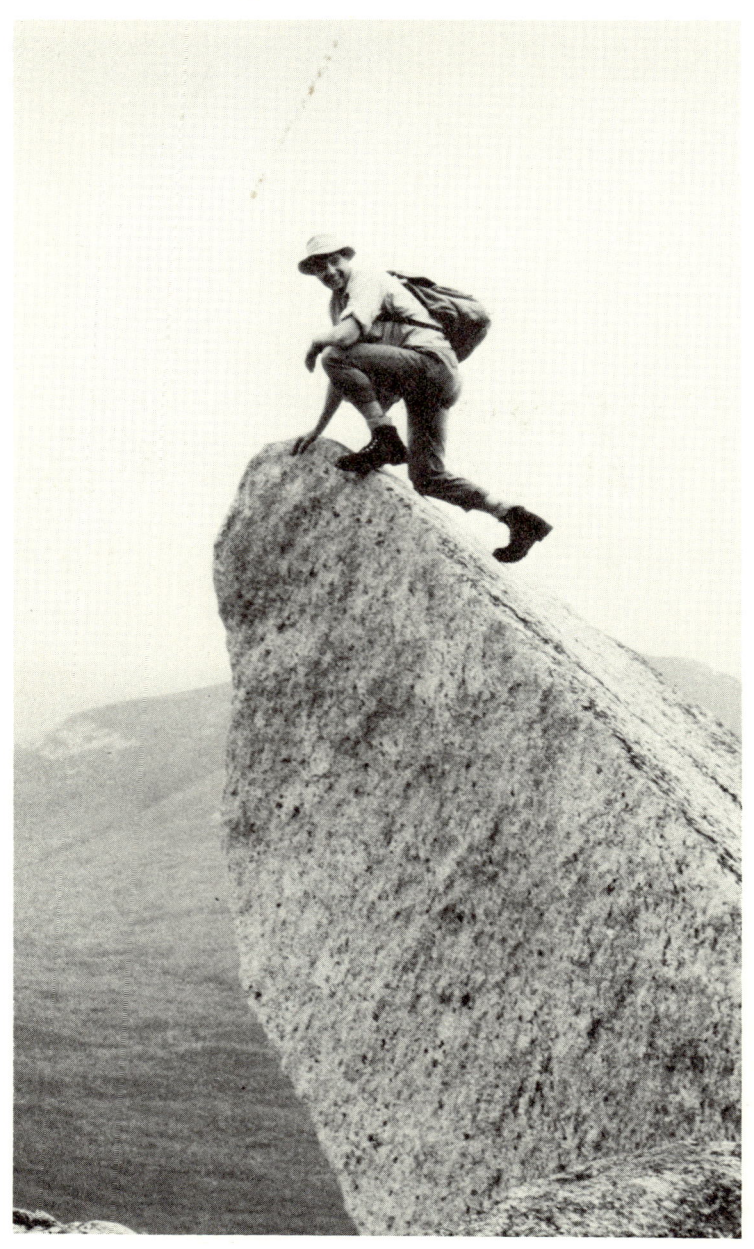

Dave Engerbretson

The Diabetic's Sports and Exercise Book

How to Play Your Way to Better Health

by JUNE BIERMANN and BARBARA TOOHEY

J. B. Lippincott Company
Philadelphia and New York

Copyright © 1977 by June Biermann and Barbara Toohey
All rights reserved
First edition
9 8 7 6 5 4 3 2 1

Printed in the United States of America

The quotation on pages 166–67 is reprinted with permission from *The Nutrition Handbook* by Carleton Fredericks, Ph.D. Copyright © 1964, all rights reserved by Major Books, Chatsworth, California.

U.S. Library of Congress Cataloging in Publication Data

Biermann, June.
    The diabetic's sports and exercise book.

    Includes index.
    1. Diabetics. 2. Exercise therapy. I. Toohey, Barbara, joint author. II. Title.
RC660.B46   616.4′62′062   76–17894
ISBN-0-397-01115-6
ISBN-0-397-01202-0 (pbk.)

To our 158 diabetic collaborators, who generously gave us their time, their experience, and their encouragement

Also by June Biermann and Barbara Toohey

THE DIABETES QUESTION AND ANSWER BOOK

under the name Margaret Bennett
BIKING FOR GROWNUPS
CROSS-COUNTRY SKIING FOR THE FUN OF IT
HOW TO SKI JUST A LITTLE BIT
THE PERIPATETIC DIABETIC
DR. OWL'S PROBLEM
FROM BAEDEKER TO WORSE
ALICE IN WOMANLAND

Contents

Foreword by O. Charles Olson, M.D.	9
Authors' Note	13
Introduction	17
1. Rx Exercise—Prescription for Diabetic Health	31
2. Shocking Experiences	57
3. Preparations and Precautions	90
4. A Mature Attitude	122
5. Significant Others	146
6. Oh, the Disadvantages of Being a Diabetic— and (Believe It or Not) Oh, the Advantages	180
Appendixes	
A. Diabetic Doers' Profiles	205
B. Blood Pressure Chart	238
C. Cholesterol and Triglycerides	239
D. Maximum Heartbeat	240
E. Chart of Calorie Expenditures	241
F. Sugar Content of Various Blood-Sugar-Raising Snacks	243
G. What School Personnel Should Know About the Student with Diabetes	245
Index	250

Foreword

The National Commission on Diabetes has recently reported that as many as ten million Americans have diabetes, known and unknown. Between 1965 and 1973 the incidence increased by over 50 percent, and diabetes now affects 5 percent of the population of the United States. At the current rate of increase—6 percent per year—the number of persons with diabetes will have doubled by the 1990s.

Because diabetes is a disorder which at the present time is controllable but not curable, the diabetic person must learn to live with it graciously and intelligently. To do this, all diabetics should avail themselves of every possible means of self-education. The first source of such education is the family physician. Most doctors, however, simply haven't the time to devote to a detailed program of instruction for every one of their diabetic patients and in many cases will refer them to a diabetic school for the in-depth understanding of the disorder that helps patient and doctor to work better together in controlling it. If a good diabetes center is not readily accessible, the next best thing is to acquire three or four good books on diabetes and not only read them but study them well.

This book is the first of its kind to be written specifically about exercise for the person with diabetes. Those of us who are in the profession of educating diabetics welcome its publication, since it fills a void that has existed too long. Of the three basic factors involved in diabetes control—diet, medication, and exercise—not nearly enough attention has been paid to the important benefits of exercise. Certainly the old idea that the physical activity of diabetics should be restricted has been abandoned, and doctors now realize that healthy diabetics are capable of, and can benefit from, vigorous exercise and participation in individual and team sports. The only important caution for the diabetic is to have a careful evaluation by his or her family physician of general physical condition and exercise tolerance before embarking on these activities—just as many nondiabetic people are advised to do. After that, the individual can decide on a specific sports and exercise program.

Diabetes control is in many respects a highly individual thing, and personal experiences with it differ. The more knowledge the diabetic has, the more successfully will he or she be able to find the best way to lead an active, healthy, and rewarding life. With this timely book, the authors have performed a real service to the diabetic population. They have spent many hours interviewing over 150 diabetic people, finding out how they enjoy and benefit from their personal exercise programs; they have talked to experts in the field of exercise physiology; and they have presented this information in a manner which all can understand and appreciate.

Readers will certainly profit by the experiences of these diabetics. They will discover how others have learned

Foreword

to cope with the problems of diet and insulin dosage and how to avoid having hypoglycemic episodes—the insulin reactions that can be such a hindrance to the diabetic sportsperson's enjoyment and success. Diabetics of all ages, as well as their parents, friends, spouses, coaches, and doctors, can be grateful for such an excellent book. I have enjoyed reading it, and I am sure they will, too.

                      O. Charles Olson, M.D., F.A.C.P.
                      Director, Diabetes Education Center
                      Director of Medical Education
                      Deaconess Hospital
                      Spokane, Washington

Authors' Note

"There are few things that offend me more than projects such as this book, whose essential premise is that I, as a diabetic, am something special and require charitable encouragement and a condescending sort of slap on the back to lift me up and convince me that I, too, can lead a normal life."

This is twenty-year-old insulin-taking-diabetic Stephen Naruk talking. Stephen has had the disease since age eight. He swims, bicycles, climbs rocks, skis—both downhill and cross country—plays tennis, and incidentally gets mad as hell at the idea that "a diabetic person is somehow especially cursed or possesses some special affliction."

We're offended, too, but not by Stephen Naruk's objection to the book we're writing. We're offended by things like the title of the *Reader's Digest* article about Philadelphia Flyer star Bobby Clarke. They called it "Hockey's Invincible Invalid," because Bobby is diabetic.

We're offended that Chicago Cubs star third baseman Ron Santo felt he had to hide his diabetes for the first five years of his major league career.

We're offended by doctors who tell their patients, as did Dave Engerbretson's when his diabetes was diagnosed at age twenty-three, "You're going to have to slow down now. Things are going to be different." At this time Dave was a college football player, track man, ski team member, and captain of the swimming team. The doctor wanted to change him into a sedentary blob. It didn't work. Now, sixteen years later, Dave is a downhill and cross-country ski instructor, backpacking and canoeing guide, camper, jogger, hunter, fly fisherman, mountain climber, spelunker, sailplane flyer, and sports-car-rallye driver. He's also managed to pick up a Ph.D. in physical education, teach at Washington State University, and become a successful free-lance outdoor writer.

We're offended when a child is diagnosed as diabetic and the parents immediately start coddling the youngster and depriving him or her of the exercise that is a basic part of the treatment of diabetes, as well as a mental-health insurance policy.

In fact, we're offended by all the free-floating misconceptions about the physical limitations of diabetics. That's why we're writing the kind of book that offends Stephen Naruk. We're determined to get rid of the ignorance and fear and prejudice and just plain nonsense about diabetes that makes this sort of book necessary. We want to prove in these pages that, as far as diabetes is concerned, the accent on the word invalid should be shifted to the second syllable, making it in-val'-id instead of in'-va-lid. This shift in emphasis changes the meaning from "sickly or disabled" to "without foundation in fact or truth"—in other words, hogwash. And we want to show how exercise and sports for diabetics of all ages and

Authors' Note

every physical condition can be a major factor in bringing that accent change about.

We feel strongly about what we say in the following pages, because diabetes is a very personal thing with us—and so are sports. The two of us have been a professional writing team for sixteen years. This is our tenth book. For eight of those years one of us—June, now age fifty-three—has been an insulin-taking diabetic. During those eight years we have published three sports books, one on downhill skiing, one on cross-country skiing, and one on bicycling, all researched equally by Barbara, the nondiabetic, and June, the diabetic. In this book, therefore, we are writing not only from our professional knowledge and experience but from our hearts, as well as from June's pancreas.

June Biermann
Barbara Toohey

Laguna Beach, California
February 1976

Introduction

The logo of the American Diabetes Association is a triangle or, if you will, a pyramid. Officially, now, the three sides represent the three major aims of the ADA: research, detection, and education. The logo, however, also harks back to an earlier ADA symbol—a triangular balance scale. This symbolic balance represented the three elements of diabetes control: diet, medication, and exercise.

Diet-medication-exercise. Even though a new logo may have replaced the old one, nothing has really changed about these basics of diabetes therapy. Prescribing the medication—insulin or pills—has always been the doctor's responsibility. The diet has been mainly in the hands of the diabetic, who, after a bit of professional guidance, has been more or less left alone to decide on an eating program. Learning about the diet hasn't been too much for most diabetics to cope with, though. Physicians and dieticians have done a great deal of work in devising eating plans and analyzing foods. To make figuring the diet easier, they've given us the Food Exchange System. In addition, there are dozens of cookbooks available, with more rattling off the presses every year. It's reached the point that you can be a *Diabetic Gourmet* and *Feast on a Diabetic Diet* if you're a *Calculating Cook*. Yes, the diabetic diet has had a lot of attention.

But what about the exercise part of the three-way diabetic balancing act? Diet-medication-exercise. Is the fact that exercise is placed last of any significance? Think back to when your diabetes was first diagnosed. You were probably immediately given one of those x-number-of-calories diet sheets that the Eli Lilly pharmaceutical company publishes. But were you also given a sheet of prescribed sets of tennis or miles of walking or swimming-pool lengths which were required of you each day? No, you weren't—because none exists. Nor did your doctor, if he was typical, analyze you and your metabolism and come up with a recommended exercise program for you.

Even if you attended one of those week-long diabetes education programs that are springing up all over the country, it's highly unlikely that one of the sessions was devoted to exercise. During the course we attended, the only time exercise was mentioned was when it was given as one of the possible reasons for an insulin reaction. ("You may have exercised a little more than usual.")

In whatever context you look at it, almost invariably the diet-medication-exercise pyramid of control has one side missing. It is our theory that this is the reason why the pyramid collapses so frequently for so many diabetics —rather than "theory," perhaps we should say "conviction," because June's personal experience is what finally taught us what it takes to keep the pyramid intact.

June has always been a very in-control diabetic. She's almost compulsive about it. She abhors the sight of the telltale color of green on her urine testing tape (Tes-Tape), because green means there's sugar in the urine and that in turn indicates there's too much sugar in the blood. She's always been willing to give up anything, certainly anything edible, to avoid that ugly green. For years she had been the very model of a well-behaved diabetic, with her doctor verbally patting her on the back at each visit.

Then came the year that we went off on a sabbatical leave of exotic travels to such legendary cities as Budapest, Prague, Vienna, Venice, and Berlin. When we got home, as the warm glow of travel experiences faded, June began to feel the cold chill of economic reality. She'd spent a lot of money and depleted her financial reserves. She was a little bit scared. But that was easy to fix, she decided. All she had to do was work harder to make up for her year of peripatetic profligacy.

So that September when the college opened, besides her regular full-time job as the college reference librarian, June signed up for some extra hours for extra pay. She took on two night shifts and an all-day Saturday stint. As life fell into place under this regime she found herself locked into a dull, rigid, grindstone-nuzzling pattern. The only day she had a breather was Sunday, which had to be given over to all the chores that had accumulated between Monday and Saturday.

June lived like this for two months. Though she ate her usual diabetic fare, she was seeing more and more green on her Tes-Tape. She started lopping items off her regular diet, but still she saw green. When she finally reported to her doctor for her bimonthly blood-sugar test, it was up to 250 (normal is around 100). This time her doctor didn't pat her on the back. In fact, he acted as if he'd like to kick her in a slightly lower spot. He made her report for a blood sugar every other day. She kept scoring over 200, even when her Tes-Tape showed yellow. It began to seem as if no amount of not eating or raising her insulin dosage would bring her score down.

It didn't take many more days for the two of us to come to a conclusion—and to our senses—and pin the blame where it belonged, on the relentless work schedule which allowed her no time for exercise.

June immediately dropped the night and Saturday assignments and went back to her evening yard work and golf-ball whapping at the driving range and to her Saturday golf and bike riding. She even started taking a one-mile walk around campus immediately after lunch every day. Her blood sugar promptly dropped back into the normal range and she was once again able to eat like a human being. That was five years ago, and she's never made that mistake since.

June's exercise story has a happy ending, but many diabetes exercise stories can't possibly end happily—because they've never even begun. Why have exercise and sports been consistently played down instead of up in the diet-medication-exercise pyramid? Part of the problem may be due to historical hangover. Before insulin was discovered, one treatment for diabetes was a near-starvation carbohydrate-free diet. The patient on this diet had to be kept inactive, because if he exercised without carbohydrates he'd have to use his own limited store of fat and protein for energy.

Even though insulin changed all that, it didn't immediately change everyone's thinking on the subject. When tennis champion Bill Talbert's diabetes was discovered when he was a fifth-grade student in 1928, he

Introduction

tried to put an optimistic face on things by telling the nurse in the hospital how his new good diet would improve his baseball playing by helping him run the bases twice as fast.

The nurse's stern reply was, "Now we can't have any of that, young man. Plenty of rest, that's what we're going to need from now on."

Historical hangover isn't the only headache, though, when it comes to getting exercise into a diabetic's life. A far greater problem is caused by the lack of information on the subject. Ask any medical library for a computer printout of the existing literature on the effect of exercise and sports on diabetes and you'll see what happens.

We had Medline, a national medical information service, run searches for us. The computer's transistorized fingers sorted through *Index Medicus* and government documents and other miscellaneous sources of medical information and came up with little more than zilch. There were a few reports about camps for diabetic children—one, written in Russian, was a study of a camp in Hungary. Another item on the list was *Keith and Tommy Climb to a New Life*, a comic book distributed by Eli Lilly and Company. Some of the articles, such as "Diabetes Mellitus in Eskimos After a Decade," appeared to have little to do with exercise. Most of the studies that were specifically involved with exercise and diabetes hardly pertained to human life situations—for example, "Metabolic and Hormonal Effects of Exercise in the Severely Streptozotocin Diabetic Rat." Only the *Scandinavian Journal of Clinical Laboratory Investigation* seemed to combine exercise and diabetes and human beings, but even it didn't give really practical advice that could be interpreted to help diabetics with their day-to-day diabetic control through exercise.

True, we have seen occasional short pieces in *Diabetes Forecast* and *Diabetes in the News* with general hints about how to use exercise to help control diabetes. We've read a number of inspirational articles in national magazines about great diabetic sportspeople like Bobby Clarke and Ron Santo. When June was first diagnosed we read Bill Talbert's *Playing for Life*, about how he made it as a diabetic tennis player in the days when exercise was considered dangerous for diabetics. But that's about all we've found to read—nothing in depth, nothing comprehensive, no guidebook or manual concerned with the important details of controlling diabetes with exercise or of practicing any sport of your choosing as either an amateur or a professional.

And yet we had had glimmerings that such information, though not in print, was available. During that same sabbatical leave referred to earlier, we had been standing in line to see the Royal Lippizan stallion rehearsals in Vienna, and we got to talking with a doctor who was in line in front of us. He was not a diabetologist, but he had a friend who had diabetes. This friend, according to the doctor, was able to control his diabetes by eating the correct diet and doing two hours of exercise a day. This allowed him to get along without insulin. At the time this sounded well nigh impossible to us, but it always stuck in our minds as something we wanted to know more about.

Another year we ran into a ski instructor who confessed to being diabetic. "But don't tell the head of the ski school," she cautioned us. "He might throw me out."

Introduction

We wondered how many diabetic ski instructors there might be—and were there diabetic members of the ski patrol too? And, if they were performing effectively, why should anyone want to throw them out or indeed have the power to do so?

Probably our most close-to-home example of the use of exercise for diabetes control was the editor of our last book on diabetes, *The Diabetes Question and Answer Book*. Shelly Lowenkopf is a lanky, wiry diabetic in his mid-forties. Since his father is an insulin-taking diabetic, he knows what's in the cards for him. Or is it? So far he doesn't take insulin; he doesn't even take pills. Insulin he considers a terrible bother to a book editor who has to sit through long editorial conferences, and the pills he believes to have the life-shortening effect that the FDA has claimed they have. That leaves him with a very strict diet and exercise (we noted at lunch that he was more strict even than June).

Shelly told us in detail about his technique for fitting two hours of exercise into his twelve-hour-a-day editing job. Every morning he arises while the chickens still have their heads under their wings and lopes off with his two dogs. By the time the sun is up he is back home and eating his calorie-calculated breakfast. Then it's off to a sedentary but safe day: diabetic fate cannot harm him, since he has that ten-mile run working on his blood sugar.

Putting together all these glimpses and glances of what exercise-oriented diabetics do, we finally figured out where the great untapped mine of information on exercise and diabetes is hidden. It is hidden inside the heads—and hearts and muscles—of diabetics. It is the mass of experience accumulated by all the diabetics who jog and run and bicycle and swim and backpack and play tennis and football and baseball and do weight lifting and karate and hang gliding. And that is where we've gone to gather the facts that all diabetics need to keep their pyramids of control from collapsing. We've gone to the diabetics—over 150 of them—who are out there Doing It.

What are these diabetics like? They are of all ages, ranging from nine to seventy-nine. They are from all the United States, including Alaska, and they are from Canada. Both sexes are represented, although (as among nondiabetics) there are more sportsmen than sportswomen. They participate in a total of seventy-four different sports, from the relatively mild walking and lawn bowling to the body-contact bone-busters like football and hockey and rugby to the sports generally not recommended for diabetics, like scuba diving and skydiving. Some have only had diabetes for a few months, but many are diabetic veterans. (Bill Talbert has had it for forty-eight years, and one woman golfer for forty-five years.) Some control their diabetes with diet, exercise, and pills, some with only diet and exercise, but the vast majority of our diabetic sportspeople are insulin takers—the very ones you'd think would be the most hesitant to engage in active sports for fear of bringing on insulin shock or receiving slow-to-heal injuries.

How did all these mines of information learn what they now know about sports and exercise for diabetics? Several give some measure of credit to their doctors. For example, one woman reports, "My doctors have taught me the basics about sports and diabetes. My first diabetic specialist taught me not to be afraid to exercise. He instilled in me the belief that exercise is very good for me

Introduction

and I should get as much as possible. . . . He gave me the general rules for exercise with diabetes."

Some mentioned that they got information from books and magazine articles—helpful, but, as one said, "too general by the time it gets into a book to actually be of much value." But over and over the theme we heard was, "I learned by experience," with such variations on that theme as "I learned on my own" and "I learned through trial and error." Even Bill Talbert, whose life has been an inspiration to so many other diabetics, learned about diabetes and sports "mostly through personal experience."

Here, then, are their personal experiences, their trials, their errors, and their ultimate successes, all woven together with the available scientific information about exercise and diabetes. We hope the resulting fabric will serve both as a security blanket and as a magic carpet for any diabetic who wants to lead an active, exciting, and healthy life.

From disease I have learned much which life could never have taught me in any other way.

—*Goethe*

The Diabetic's Sports and Exercise Book

1

Rx Exercise—
Prescription for Diabetic Health

Dave Engerbretson, the diabetic professor of physical education at Washington State, is one of the few researchers who have ever devised an experiment to study the use of regular exercise to control diabetes. He actually conducted two separate studies, one in 1962 at the University of Illinois and another in 1970 at Penn State.

In the first study three insulin-taking college men exercised for one hour six days a week. Three days a week they did running and calisthenics and two days weight training and jogging. On weekends they were asked to stay active in whatever sports they preferred. After six weeks of this program their required insulin dosage had dropped an average of 17 units. This is particularly dramatic when you stop to consider that, although severe diabetics can take over 50 units of insulin a day, moderate diabetics get by on 20 to 50 units and mild diabetics usually take under 20 units. One student put the cherry on the insulin-drop sundae by going off insulin entirely for the last three weeks of the program.

In spite of the decreased insulin dosage, the average blood sugar of these men also dropped. At the beginning it was 220 (80 to 120 is normal) and at the end it was 115. The conclusion of the study was that regular physical exercise did indeed produce an improvement in diabetes control.

In the second study five insulin-dependent college men jogged thirty to forty-five minutes five days a week for fourteen weeks. The result was the same as in the first study: Both the insulin dosage and the blood sugar dropped. So again Dave had shown that regular physical exercise improves diabetes control.

Dr. O. Charles Olson, Director of the Diabetes Education Center of the Deaconess Hospital in Spokane, Washington, came to a similar conclusion on the basis of his twenty-seven years' experience taking care of diabetics: "It is very obvious to those of us who have observed diabetics in *sustained* athletic endeavors that insulin requirements will go down as much as 50 to 60 percent even with concurrent increase in carbohydrate intake."

Many of our diabetic sports enthusiasts have experienced similar insulin reductions as a result of their own exercise activities. When we asked if they'd been able to cut back or eliminate any medication because of exercise, almost to a man—and woman—they answered that they had decreased their insulin by one tenth, one fourth, one half, or even, as in the case of TV's Dan Rowan, two thirds. (This dramatic drop of Rowan's happens when he escapes from the long hours of stress and confinement of his performing life for an active, outdoor, tennis-every-day vacation at his Florida retreat.) One diabetic even had an off-again, on-again tale to tell:

"When I first realized my diabetic condition I was taking 27 units of NPH insulin. At the time I was living in Florida and active all the time. With diet and exercise I was able to cut down my insulin intake to 5 units. I asked the doctor if I could try Orinase [a blood-sugar-lowering pill] because of the small dosage of insulin. It worked as long as I was active, but I went to college in Vermont six months after switching and quit exercising for four years. After one year on Orinase and no exercise I had to go back to insulin. The four-year period without exercise adversely affected my condition. I had to take more insulin, to the point that now I am taking two shots per day. Since taking up cycling, however, my condition is stable and all is under control."

INVISIBLE INSULIN

Considering these testimonials, it wouldn't be an exaggeration to call exercise a form of "invisible insulin." Although it isn't literally insulin, it has the same effect as insulin. This is why—if you are one of those diabetics who inject insulin to help control your diabetes—you also have to estimate how much "invisible insulin" you're giving yourself when exercising, and then you either have to eat more to compensate for it or take less injected insulin. Otherwise, your invisible insulin will pull your blood sugar down below normal.

How insulin and/or exercise perform this feat of lowering the blood sugar is something of a mystery even to biochemists. The form of sugar in the blood is glucose, and it's this glucose that the cells burn for energy. Insulin somehow opens the cell gates and lets the glucose in. Exercise acts as a kind of booster to insulin, making less of it necessary—just as Dave Engerbretson proved in his two studies.

We've only come across one case in which a diabetic's insulin requirement went up with exercise, and this was because of the sports objective of the diabetic. Joe Brink of Cincinnati deliberately and consciously increased his insulin dosage, because he wanted to eat more and put on weight. Joe is now famous as the weight-lifting and body-building enthusiast who in 1973 won the title of Mr. Cincinnati. In four years, according to his wife, he went "from a 130-pound weakling to a 200-pound tower of strength." To add this much weight he increased his insulin dosage by 10 units daily to cover the extra calories needed to gain the weight.

So Joe's insulin went up to achieve his goal, but, as we've seen, the usual thing is for insulin needs to go down with exercise. Why is it desirable for insulin needs to go down? First, the less insulin you inject, the less are your chances of having to cope with insulin shock. Then—and this is definitely a consideration in these days of economic crisis—it just plain costs a lot less if you don't have to shoot as much insulin. The cost of insulin, like the cost of everything else, is climbing. If you can cut back on insulin, it will help you at least stay even on your insulin expense account.

KICK THE NEEDLE?

You may have been as intrigued as we were by the thought of going off insulin entirely, as did one of the subjects in Dave's experiments and as did the Florida exercise enthusiast who went onto Orinase. It is an intriguing thought—no needles, no fear of insulin reactions. As one teenager says of insulin taking, "It's a super-drag!"

But it is—for most of us, unfortunately—also a super-necessity.

June takes only around 15 units a day, so we logically thought—from reading the studies of an average insulin drop of 17 units during a vigorous daily exercise program—that she might be one of the lucky ones who, with exercise, could give up insulin entirely. She tried a one-hour-a-day calisthenics and jogging program. It didn't work for her. The only time, in fact, in her entire history of diabetes that she was ever able to go off insulin for even one day and suffer no spilling (sugar in the urine) was once when she was doing a full day of ski touring. And it's a little hard to ski-tour all day every day and still conduct a life on the side, to say nothing of finding sufficient snow.

She complained of this failure to Dick Bernstein, a New York corporate officer by trade, a weight lifter by sport, and one of the most knowledgeable diabetics we know (by virtue of his own intelligence and the fact that his wife is a doctor). These are Dick's comments on the subject of eliminating the need for insulin with a regular exercise program:

"Earlier in this century—before the advent of commercially available insulin and perhaps even before that—a combination of exercise and a starvation diet were the standard treatment for diabetes mellitus. The great bulk of people thus treated did not survive.

"The starvation diet was truly a starvation diet and the people became very thin and weak and the exercise routine was practically roadwork. It was grueling and laborious and took many hours each day. In fact, from what I read, many years ago the bulk of the patient's time would have to be devoted to his exercise.

"I'd be surprised to hear that any juvenile-onset diabetics survived this regimen. I gather that June is a maturity-onset case, but I certainly wouldn't expect her to be able to eliminate her insulin entirely. I would certainly expect a dropoff in insulin requirements."

The final word on the relationship of exercise to insulin requirements came to us out of the Elliott P. Joslin Research Laboratory of the Harvard Medical School. According to Dr. Leo Krall, editor of *Diabetes Forecast*, Dr. Neil Ruderman "is one of the few people who have done actual research in this area." Here are Dr. Ruderman's conclusions:

> It has long been appreciated that exercise can lower blood glucose and diminish the requirement for insulin in the diabetic. Less appreciated is the fact that some insulin is needed for this to occur. A patient with insulin-requiring diabetes may actually increase his blood glucose and even precipitate ketosis [acid poisoning] if he exercises vigorously without taking his insulin. There appear to be two reasons for this:
>
> 1. A small amount of insulin is required for exercise to stimulate glucose transport into muscle. (Berger, Hagg and Ruderman, *Biochem. J.* 146:231, 1975.)
>
> 2. In the absence of insulin, glucose production by the liver, which even in nondiabetic individuals is increased during exercise, may become excessive. (Vranic, Kovacevic and Wrenshall, *Fed. Proc.* 29: 314, 1970.)
>
> Thus although exercise has many potentially beneficial effects in the diabetic . . . it is not a substitute for insulin.

PANDORA'S PILLBOX

Those of you who are among the 1½ million diabetics who take their medication in the form of pills may be wondering at this point if exercise might make it possible for you to stop taking your Orinase or D.B.I. or whatever. And well you should be wondering, because there's been a lot of talk and writing lately about the dangers of oral hypoglycemic agents, as the doctors call them. The concern over pills began when the results of an eight-year study by researchers revealed more cardiovascular disease among pill takers than among diabetics controlled by either diet alone or by diet and insulin.

Many diabetes specialists question the validity of this study. Even so, the federal Food and Drug Administration takes it seriously enough to consider requiring labels on the pills to warn that their prolonged use could increase a person's risk of death by heart disease. Some doctors have stopped prescribing pills; many have not. In short, if at this moment you could ask for a collective medical opinion as to whether or not these pills will shorten your life, you'd get a firm unequivocal maybe.

We are certainly not presumptuous enough to claim that we have the definitive answer to this controversy. We are, however, willing to say what we'd do if we were pill-taking diabetics. We'd do everything in our power (and willpower) to see if we could control our diabetes by a rigid adherence to diet and a *very* regular exercise program. From our observation it seems that diet plus exercise is far more likely to take a person off pills than to take a person off insulin. Many diabetics, we feel, tend to use the pills as an easy way out, a way to avoid being careful in their diets and regular in their exercise routines. It's like the way others in our pill-popping society prefer to take tranquilizers rather than make the tremendous effort needed to solve the problems that make tranquilizers necessary.

June feels so strongly about drugs that she would not go onto pills, even if she could use them as a substitute for insulin—even if they eventually should regain their former approved status. Insulin is a natural body hormone, while the oral hypoglycemics are drugs—foreign substances you put into your body—and all drugs, even "harmless" ones like good old aspirin, have some kind of detrimental side effect. Our advice, then, to you pill takers is to discuss with your doctor whether or not he thinks you might be able to handle your diabetes with diet and exercise alone. Exercise just may be the only hypoglycemic agent you need. And it is not only an invisible drug but one with only beneficial side effects.

THE WEIGHING GAME

The French classify diabetics into two groups, *les maigres* (the leans) and *les gras* (the fats). In some ways this is better than our usual way of classifying diabetics as juvenile-onset and maturity-onset, because regardless of the age of onset most lean diabetics have to use insulin and most fat ones don't. Dr. Ralph Alexander, president of the Northern California Diabetes Association, in his paper "Ski and Après-Ski with Diabetes," also prefers to put diabetics into lean and fat categories.

In most cases the lean insulin-taking diabetics have trouble putting and keeping weight on, while the fat ones have the problem of taking and keeping it off. Oddly enough, exercise helps both classifications with their problem. How can this be? How can exercise be all things to all diabetics?

Well, let's take the fats first. Exercise has long been known to be one of the ways of losing weight. Putting it simply, you lose weight when you burn up more calories than you eat, and exercising obviously burns off more calories than lounging around does. Therefore, an overweight diabetic who exercises and does not increase his eating burns off calories and loses weight. That's not too hard to fathom.

But why does exercise have the opposite effect on the leans? How is it that they can put on weight by exercising? The answer is that with exercise the leans stay in better control and their food is totally utilized by the body instead of being thrown out and wasted as sugar in the urine. Also, when glucose from the diet cannot be adequately utilized, the body starts eating itself up, a kind of do-it-yourself cannibalism. Here's the experience of Dave Engerbretson: "I'm a rather lean, muscular 180–185 pounds. If I don't exercise I lose weight when my control is affected and my sugar levels increase. I then must return to my high activity level to gain it back."

A Maryland high school football tight end and linebacker told us he has noticed the same thing: "The more I exercise the lower my sugar stays and the lower my sugar stays the more weight I gain."

Then, of course, there's Mr. Cincinnati, with his 70-pound weight gain in four years. To accomplish this he did a systematic two-hour workout in his gym six days a week and ate approximately 5,000 calories a day. He says he has little fat on him. He's mostly muscle.

Here we might mention another reason why exercise causes an increase of weight in relatively thin but athletic diabetics. It's the simple fact that muscle weighs more than fat. But as the *Royal Canadian Air Force Exercise Plans for Physical Fitness* book points out, "This muscle weight is useful weight and will improve the way you look and feel." A moving man we once met was about six feet tall and weighed 205 pounds, yet he looked as skinny as a greyhound. The guy was nothing but skin-covered muscle, as he vividly demonstrated by single-handedly hefting king-sized sofas and a giant antique buffet so heavy it could hardly be pushed, let alone picked up, by a normal man. (The very useful R.C.A.F. book can, by the way, be purchased for $1.25; it's published by Pocket Books.)

TIGHTWIRE ACT

An insulin-taking diabetic, according to Dave Engerbretson, "walks a tightwire between high blood sugar on one side and low blood sugar on the other. He starts to teeter one way and he's got to eat something, and he starts to teeter the other way and he's got to get some exercise or take some more insulin, and he's constantly hurrying through life trying to keep from falling off his wire."

In this respect, exercise can again come to the rescue. It can, in effect, turn the wire into a board with lots more room to walk on and much less risk of falling off one side or the other. A Pittsburgh businessman, diabetic since his early thirties, sums it up like this: "Exercise, particularly bicycling, which I participate in more frequently, weather permitting, than golf or skiing, helps to maintain my blood sugar at a more even level. When I don't get much exercise I have a greater tendency to have wide swings in blood-sugar level from very high to very low within a few hours' time."

Again, exercise appears to be almost magical. How can the same activity prevent both high blood sugar with spilling in the urine and low blood sugar with insulin reactions? The first half of this stabilizing effect of exercise we've already discussed when we showed you how exercise works as "invisible insulin" to prevent high blood-sugar levels by helping glucose get into the cells. The process by which exercise does the opposite—prevents low blood-sugar levels—involves some rather complex body chemistry. We'll try to explain it without being as simplistic as a TV commercial for a headache remedy or as abstruse as Professor Irwin Corey.

You remember we said earlier that glucose is the fuel used by body cells. What we didn't say was that the body has a way to store glucose for future use. What happens is that, when excess glucose is available, our interior chemical factory converts the excess to a complex form of sugar called glycogen. Glycogen, or "animal starch," can be reconverted to glucose whenever the body is low on that fuel. The breakdown of glycogen to glucose is known as glycogenolysis.

Glycogen is manufactured and stored by both liver cells and muscle cells. The glycogen stored in the liver can be turned back to glucose and sent into the bloodstream to literally save your life in an extreme insulin shock. The glycogen stored in the muscles can be turned into glucose again to provide fuel for the muscles during low-blood-sugar periods. There is even a special way that, with sustained exercise, the muscles can help the liver manufacture glycogen (this process is called the lactic acid cycle).

All in all, the total amount of glycogen stored in the liver and muscles is about enough to support the body's energy needs for one day. This means that with enough insulin and/or exercise to help the body deposit its normal stores of glycogen, a diabetic can count on having an ample internal reserve of glucose available for hypoglycemic emergencies. And that's how, as Dick Bernstein puts it, "Exercise literally helps you coming and going."

Furthermore, exercise doesn't merely affect your blood sugar for an hour or two, or until the clock strikes midnight on the day you've exercised. No, there's a lingering or holdover effect that many diabetics have become aware of. A woman who is active in no less than five different vigorous sports says, "Exercise tends to lower my blood sugar level in general for the rest of the day and the beginning of the next day, not just during the period when I am actually doing the exercising. . . . I have to be prepared for an insulin reaction during the night. Exercising vigorously seems to 'loosen up' my whole system in that it brings a complete lowering of my blood sugar for the whole day and into the next." Other active diabetics agree. As one cyclist and tennis player says, "The increased need for food sometimes catches up with me the next morning about eleven A.M. when that day's insulin is working on a lower sugar level from the day before."

Still another physically active diabetic says, "I usually have my most severe reactions the day after a day of strenuous activity. Mondays are the most critical day because of extra activities over the weekend. I have had more reactions on Monday than any other day."

Our executive weight lifter, Dick Bernstein, capitalizing on this holdover effect, has designed for himself an exercise routine that varies from day to day over a five-day cycle. One day he concentrates on leg exercises, another day he concentrates on arm exercises, and another day on chest exercises, and so on. Dick says that, by developing masses of muscle that are in regular states of activity in this way, the effect for him is almost as if he were receiving insulin in small amounts all day long.

Then there are men like the University of Minnesota chemistry professor and long-distance runner who runs 5 to 10 miles *every single day* plus an occasional 26.2-mile marathon. Professor Edward Leete has such marvelous blood glucose stability that he has virtually given up testing his urine for sugar. When he does, he finds it is usually only between 0.1 percent and 0.5 percent, which is a kind of long-distance record in itself, considering that Leete has been diabetic for seventeen years and takes 50 units of insulin a day. His diabetes is so stable that he visits his physician only once a year "to show her how healthy I am."

THE HEART OF THE MATTER

In matters of disease, diabetes is known as "the great complicator." What happens to the so-called normal person usually happens more so to a diabetic—especially an out-of-control diabetic.

Probably the most dramatic health happening in the United States in recent years has been the increase in cardiovascular problems. A whole new vocabulary has come into prominence:

Arteriosclerosis—thickening and hardening of the arteries

Atherosclerosis—a form of arteriosclerosis in which fatlike substances are deposited on the inner layer of the arteries.
Cholesterol—a fatlike substance in the blood
Hypertension—high blood pressure
Triglycerides—blood fats

Thanks to our modern sedentary way of life and the advanced technology of our food industry, the average person is more and more susceptible to these problems. What are the recommendations to prevent them? First, a diet that is a ringer for the low-animal-fat, low-cholesterol diabetic diet. And, second, what else but good old exercise?

According to Dr. Lenore Zohman, an internationally known exercise physiologist and physician, exercise training reduces risk of heart attack by lowering both blood pressure and heart rate, by lowering the triglyceride level and temporarily the cholesterol level, by improving the way the body handles carbohydrates, by decreasing the body's secretion of the "adrenaline-type" chemical it produces in response to emotional stress, and by changing the clotting power of the blood so that it is less likely that a clot will form.

A diabetic can get the same cardiovascular advantages as everyone else—plus more. He also gets the advantage of keeping his diabetes in better control, and in-control diabetics generally have lower cholesterol and triglyceride levels than out-of-control ones do. Dick Bernstein's story, for instance, is pretty convincing:

"When I started off in 1968 with my exercises I had been running a cholesterol level of approximately 300 for a number of years. Now in 1968 I was thirty-four years old. For a thirty-four-year-old man to have a cholesterol of 300 is a grossly abnormal condition. After the first year or so of these exercise routines my cholesterol dropped to approximately 175. My cholesterol levels sometimes even go as low as 145. And now I'm forty-one years old, and to speak of a forty-one-year-old diabetic with a cholesterol level of 145—and when you're talking juvenile-onset diabetes, yet—you have a situation that's almost hard to believe. Yet it can be documented by my doctor's records." Dick also sports a triglyceride level of 105.

Probably the most convincing figures we've seen about what exercise does for keeping the body out of cardiovascular trouble come from that long-distance runner, Professor Leete. At the age of forty-six he weighs 145 pounds, just as he did twenty-eight years ago when he was eighteen. His blood pressure is 120/75, that of a young

Chemistry professor and runner Edward Leete (left) has the right formula for diabetes health.

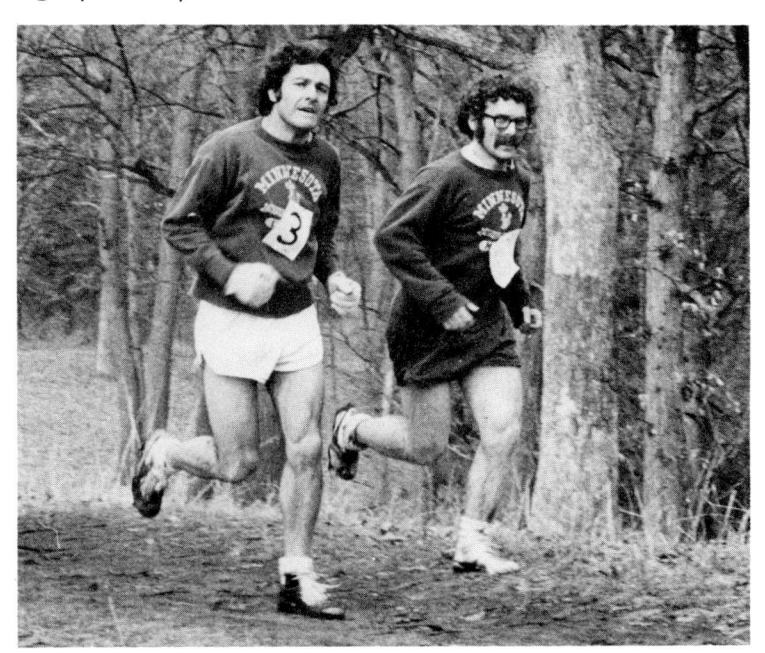

man. His cholesterol level is a low 140, and his triglyceride level is 115. His resting heartbeat is a low 55 and his maximum heartbeat at exhaustion is 175, which is the best possible for his age group. Small wonder that Leete believes that "the long-distance runner will inherit the earth. He will live longer, he will never have a heart attack, he will remain mentally alert till his nineties. He will probably die by being hit by a truck!"

You can see from this that, if diabetes is the great complicator, exercise can be the great uncomplicator for diabetics. (If you want to check Bernstein's and Leete's figures—and your own—against the normal range, see appendixes B, C, and D.)

THE HUNGRY YOU

The complaint we most often hear from adult-onset diabetics who don't have to take insulin is, "I just don't get enough to eat on my diet. I'm always hungry." Apropos of this, Dr. Jean Mayer of Harvard, writing about weight problems, once made a succinct statement that we have always cherished. "You have three choices: you can exercise more, or you can always be hungry, or you can be fat."

He was, of course, not speaking about diabetics. He was speaking about the majority of the sedentary adult American population. A maturity-onset diabetic has only *two* choices. The choice of being fat is eliminated because if you're fat, you're leaving yourself open to the manifold cardiovascular complications of diabetes. To put it bluntly, fat could turn out to be your personal padding for an early coffin.

Rx Exercise—Prescription for Diabetic Health 47

Your two choices, then, are to exercise more or to diet and always be hungry. Actually, if you look at it logically, the choice should be a fairly easy one to make. After all, exercise, if it is in the form of some sport you enjoy, is a pleasure with many physically and emotionally beneficial side effects, while always being hungry is never anything but a rotten condition to live with. Why not choose the double pleasure of exercising and eating more?

We just received by telepathy your counterclaim that exercise won't do you one bit of good with your hunger problem, because exercise makes you so enormously and ravenously hungry that either you'll gulp down so much food you'll wind up putting on more weight than ever or else you'll feel hungrier than ever.

This is an old saw that new nutritionists like Dr. Mayer have taken the teeth out of. They've done experiments with both mice and men and the results have always been the same. To quote Dr. Mayer, "The subjects with regular moderate activity ate somewhat less (and were considerably thinner) than the inactive subjects!"

Putting it in mouse terms, when Dr. Mayer made formerly sedentary obese mice run a treadmill for from twenty minutes to an hour a day, they ate less and they lost weight. Incidentally, given the results of these experiments plus others he had done earlier, Dr. Mayer concluded that people who lose their weight through exercise tend to keep it off better than those who lose it by dieting.

Now, of course, this doesn't mean that, for example, a high school football player in the midst of football season doesn't eat more to maintain the same weight than he eats in the off-season, when he's not practicing and playing his sport regularly. He does eat more during football season, quite a lot more. What we—and Dr. Mayer—are referring to are the very sedentary types as compared to those who are moderately but regularly active.

If you're a sedentary maturity-onset diabetic, then, exercise can make it possible for you to not be hungry in two ways: You'll be able to eat more because of the calories you've burned off, yet your hunger will be more easily assuaged. Here we have still another of the seemingly magical contradictions of exercise.

EAT AND GROW THIN

With the insulin takers the problem is not so much one of getting fat but one of staying in control. If you overeat all the time, the body is not able to metabolize the excessive glucose your overeating has produced. As a consequence, your blood sugar soars and your urine becomes as sweet as the Lemonade River that flows in the Big Rock Candy Mountain.

June once decided that this would be a great way for an insulin-taking diabetic to drop a few pounds. All you'd do is lower your insulin a little and eat all you wanted of anything you wanted. Only the amount of food your insulin could escort into the cells would be used, she figured. The rest would just be flushed down the toilet and you'd lose weight.

She made the mistake of offering this keen reducing theory to her doctor. This caused *him* to flush—and blanch and turn several other colors. Only a moment's reflection will show why. The basic flaw with this reducing scheme is that you would be running around all the time with sky-

Rx Exercise—Prescription for Diabetic Health 49

high blood sugar. And what does constant high blood sugar do? It gives you all those diabetic complications of legend and song: cardiovascular and kidney disasters, blindness, gangrene, diabetic coma, and—well, you know the rest, including rest in peace.

But insulin takers are not doomed to a starvation diet, or even to an abnormal one. Did you know there are diabetics who stay in excellent control but who "eat almost anything"? One of these is the aforementioned Professor Leete, and here's a sample of what he typically stows away in a day.

> Breakfast: grapefruit sections, cereal with milk and raisins, slice of bread, a boiled egg, coffee
> Lunch: soup, meat sandwich, canned fruit, milk
> Dinner: meat, potatoes, peas or other vegetable, apple pie and ice cream, milk, coffee

And just to add insult to injury, he tells us, "I often have a beer before dinner, plus cheese and crackers."

Now, don't misinterpret us; we're not advocating *this* diet for you (unless, of course, like Professor Leete you run ten miles a day and run them in an hour flat). No, we're only demonstrating that the more constantly and strenuously you exercise, the more normally you can eat. Over and over again we've heard comments like these from sports-dedicated diabetics: "I can eat almost anything while skiing"; "I eat a regular diet and I don't count calories"; "I have a free diet."

Even usually verboten foods can be indulged in by insulin takers who are schussing the ski slopes or biking uphill or against twenty-mile winds—indeed, they are often necessary. When June is cross-country skiing she can sit down at noon and eat a stevedore-style lunch without counting exchanges or calories. It's almost like being a nondiabetic. (Incidentally, according to Dr. Grant Gwinup of the University of California at Irvine Medical School, the highest energy expenditure ever measured in exercise that can be sustained for only an hour or less was recorded in cross-country skiers. They burned up 1,300 calories per hour.)

For adult-onset diabetics of normal weight who maintain control without insulin or pills, exercise of the good-rolling-sweat variety can burn up so many calories that they, too, can have larger portions and more variety and they can leave the table feeling full to the gills instead of hollow.

THE HAPPY HORMONE

Almost every diabetic has at one time or another seen how one's mental health affects the disease. Mental or emotional stress is known to trigger the onset of diabetes. Stress is recognized as a potent factor in upsetting control.

How can exercise help in this area? Exercise simply makes you feel better. It may be just escaping from the pressure-cooker situation you're caught up in for a while. And then again it may be the releasing of "the happy hormone," norepinephrine. A British medical team headed by Dr. Malcolm Carruthers found that only ten minutes of exercise was enough to double the body's level of norepinephrine and make a person's spirits rise.

Professor Leete keeps his happy hormone level perennially high with his hour-a-day ten-mile run and says, "I am mentally alert and not depressed like many of my colleagues who have succumbed to 'middle age.'"

Rx Exercise—Prescription for Diabetic Health

Dr. Ethan Sims and his wife, in their "Dialogue About Diabetes and Exercise" in the *ADA Forecast* for July–August 1974, quoted one of their friends describing his exercise experience:

> I also experience a type of "high" which has not often been commented on. The initial exhaustion of a run wears off in about five to ten minutes. About a half hour later, a gentle warmth begins to suffuse the lower limbs which complements a state of complete physical relaxation. The sensorium is sharpened and thinking becomes more acute. A total sense of well-being which may last three to four hours permeates the event.

Lynn Caine, the (nondiabetic) author of *Widow*, explained how she used exercise to help her make it through the night during the early, most painful stages of her widowhood.

> The first thing I learned was "move the body." It sounds so simple, but it works. Now when panic struck in the night, I would tell myself, "move the body." It took tremendous effort, but I forced myself out of bed and onto the floor to do exercises. "You only have to do ten," I would tell myself, "but do them. Move the body. One and two and three and . . ." It helped a lot. Then I bought a stationary exercise bicycle. That was even better. Get over to the bicycle and pedal twenty-five revolutions. That got the blood going and immediately I felt a little better.

In our own dismal periods we've experienced the cheering effects of exercise. And if we weren't convinced before working on this book of the mental-health values of exercise, we are now. All the diabetic sportspeople we've been in contact with are the most upbeat and positive and optimistic people we've ever met. There's not a grouch or a self-pitier in the pack. As we'll explain later, many of them not only don't consider diabetes a handicap, they consider it in some ways an advantage. You can hardly get more upbeat and positive and optimistic than that!

THE FUN FACTOR

So far we may have made exercise sound like a medication, a treatment, a bitter pill that must be swallowed to produce good physical and mental health for diabetics. But exercise can be taken in the form of sports, and sports, along with the health benefits derived from them, are also fun and games. Someone once aptly called sports "the toy department of life." A diabetic definitely should not deprive himself of the joys of this department.

Just which sports joys are in the realm of possibility for a diabetic? Every one of them. Here's a list of the sports practiced by the diabetics we contacted:

archery	canoeing
backpacking	cross-country running
badminton	cross-country skiing
baseball	diving
basketball	downhill skiing
bicycling	field hockey
boating	fishing
body building	folk dancing
body surfing	football
bowling	gliding
boxing	golf
calisthenics	gymnastics
camping	handball

hiking	running
hockey	sailing
horseback riding	sailplanes
hunting	scuba diving
ice fishing	show jumping
ice hockey	skin diving
ice skating	skydiving
isometrics	snowshoeing
jogging	soccer
jumping rope	softball
karate	spelunking
kayaking	sportscar rallying
lawn bowling	squash
motocross	surfing
motorcycling	swimming
mountain climbing	tennis
paddleball	tobogganing
Ping-Pong	track
platform tennis	tumbling
pool	volleyball
rock climbing	walking
rodeo	waterskiing
rollerskating	weight lifting
rowing	wrestling

As you can see, hardly any sport is left out. Any sport that is not included—we don't have, for example, anyone who's addicted to lacrosse or logrolling—is missing simply because either it's not commonly practiced or because we just happened not to be in contact with a diabetic who did it. Since, as we mentioned previously, many diabetics indulge in sports that are sometimes not recommended for them—like scuba diving or skydiving—it's clear that diabetics can and *do* do everything.

One counsel we can give you is to choose a sport you

love. That's what almost all the diabetics we talked to did. When we asked if diabetes had anything to do with their choice of a sport, we got answers like:

"My diabetes has no influence on me, for I do not consider it anything that should be catered to."

"I have never really thought about my diabetes having any effect on what I do. I like track and basketball and feel I have a little bit of talent in those areas, whereas I would love to be a gymnast, but I feel I don't have it in me to do it."

"It didn't actually make a difference. I got diabetes when I was five and grew like almost any other kid."

"I generally do what I like doing, and if my diabetes poses a problem to my participation in the sport, or vice versa, I straighten it out."

Only the weight lifters like Dick Bernstein and Joe Brink, it seems, took up their sport as much or more for therapy as for pleasure.

One last piece of advice came to us from Bill Talbert, who chose tennis at least partially because it's a "sport of a lifetime." He's right. It is very wise to include among your sports interests those activities you can enjoy (and gain diabetic benefits from) through the years after your physical-contact team sports days are behind you. It's also a good idea to select some sports that don't require a whole gang of other people to play with you.

PEOPLE WHO NEED SPORTSPEOPLE

One of the best reasons for a diabetic to get involved in sports is the opportunity for meeting new friends. New friends, of course, are always welcome, but sports friends have a special value for a diabetic.

In the first place, what you do with these friends when you get together with them is not only fun but healthy. You may not have noticed it, but in most social circles the major pastimes when friends get together are drinking and eating and sitting around talking. This is especially true in the middle-aged group when maturity-onset diabetes is in flower. June complains that all of her friends entertain in the same way—before-dinner drinks and conversation, a long, lingering dinner with wine and conversation, followed by liqueurs and more conversation. They can stretch all this out to five or six hours.

Eating and drinking to that extent is disastrous for a diabetic, and, while conversation isn't harmful in itself, just sitting around all evening moving nothing more than your jaws is definitely not part of the diabetic regime.

Another reason why sportspeople make good friends is that most of them have at least some interest in taking care of themselves, keeping their weight down, eating the right kinds of foods, and getting enough sleep. It's a lot easier to remember to take care of your own health when those around you aren't abusing theirs—and egging you on to do the same.

"Just a little piece of pecan pie can't hurt you."

"Aw, c'mon, you can have half a drink more."

"Going home? Why, it's only a little after midnight. We're just getting started. Don't be a party pooper."

Far better to hear friends say:

"No, I'd better pass on the pie. I'm trying to get rid of five pounds so I'll be in shape for the ski season."

"Just give me a diet soda. I'm in training."

"I guess I'd better hit the hay. I've got an early golf starting time tomorrow."

Of course, you're not always home safe if you become deeply involved with sports and hang around with sportspeople. You just might become a star and be subjected to that unique form of sedentary confinement and gastronomic torture known as "the banquet." One of the few negative statements you hear coming out of Ron Santo's mouth is, "I *hate* banquets."

2

Shocking Experiences

The main and constant worry for insulin-taking diabetics is that they will go into what is variously known as insulin shock, an insulin reaction, hypoglycemia, or low blood sugar. Reactions are especially worrisome because they cause a loss of control over mind and body. The brain and central nervous system burn blood glucose primarily for their fuel. Reactions happen when these crucial cell collections run out of glucose. Then it's good-bye motor control and hello vagueness, confusion, irritability, erratic behavior, and in the later stages, convulsions and unconsciousness. Ultimately, and fortunately very rarely, there can be death. According to Dr. O. Charles Olson, "Death from hypoglycemia is very likely brain death, but no matter how it occurs it is still final!"

When we began gathering information for this book we figured that diabetics who are active in sports would have an excessive number of these reactions. It seemed it would be particularly difficult to eat just the right amount of food and take just the right amount of insulin to cover the amount of exercise. Consequently, we asked these sports-minded diabetics to describe their most dramatic and memorable incidents of insulin shock in order to help other diabetics avoid such happenings. We were amazed by their answers. In many cases the most dramatic incidents occurred *not* on the football field or tennis court or in a gym or any other area where sports are practiced, but in much more safe and tranquil-seeming places.

Weight lifter Joe Brink wins the humdinger prize for a shocking-experience double-header. It happened in, of all places, a hospital.

Joe was hospitalized for an infected foot. He had stepped on a nail when he was remodeling his garage into a gym. The foot was to be operated on in order to drain it. On the day before the operation, thanks to low blood sugar, Joe was found sitting nude on the over-the-bed table quacking like a duck. (He said he bet we'd never heard that one before, and we had to agree!)

Then, after the operation when he was in a lot of pain and it was anguish even to lower his foot, he was discovered in a deep state of hypoglycemia trotting around the corridors on the newly operated-on extremity, apparently feeling no pain.

Joe attributes these reactions to the fact that his surgery took place at a hospital where his regular diabetologist didn't practice. His family doctor, who was not as familiar with Joe's diabetes, was directing the insulin dosage.

Dick Bernstein's most memorable reaction took place in his office at work. He considers it his most memorable, because while he was in his low-blood-sugar state he quit his job.

One seventeen-year-old diabetic still remembers a reaction that took place in the ninth grade. "I was taking a math test right before lunch. I began to feel strange so I ate some jelly beans. However, I guess those were not enough for I did very poorly on the test and when I began looking it over the next day I knew how to do the problems but did not even remember taking the test."

The moral here is that insulin reactions can happen anywhere, and shunning sports and exercise is no guarantee of leading a nonshock diabetic life. In fact, when you come right down to it, there is no way for an insulin-taking diabetic to totally avoid occasional hypoglycemic incidents, short of spilling heavily all the time—a condition which carries with it its own set of destructive hazards. As one of the diabetic clichés puts it, reactions are the price you pay for good control. The sports-minded diabetic, however, does have the advantage of the stabilizing effect of exercise working for him—and he can keep his reactions infrequent and can learn to head them off in their early stages.

BALANCING ACT

Roger C. Larson, a registered physical therapist and professor in the Department of Physical Education at Washington State University, has spent the last five years working with over 150 adult diabetics trying to get them started on an exercise program. He has perfected a technique for getting any diabetic of any age into any sport with minimal reaction risk.

"Do whatever you like to do," is his advice, "but do something that you can be consistent with and something that you can measure. In other words, if you like swimming, get to a place where you can swim twenty to twenty-five laps and see how this sets with you. Find out. Do something that you can measure. If you're a person that likes to cycle—all right, cycle, but cycle a specific distance at a specific rate of speed for a specific time so you can measure it and adjust your insulin and food accordingly. Get a balance there."

Besides getting the balance that Roger Larson speaks of when you work into your sport this way, you get something else: a knowledge of your body and how it reacts to specific amounts of exercise. You have to learn this about your own body. Strict rules just can't apply.

Ron Santo realized this when his diabetes was diagnosed at age eighteen. At the time he was at a rookie training camp just getting started in professional baseball. He couldn't just guess about how his body was going to function during a game. He had to *know*. He had to *know* what the warning signals for a reaction are. He had to *know* how long he had from the first sign until the reaction really hit. He had to *know* what would bring him out of a reaction and how long it would take to do it. Santo's solution was to take a good supply of sugar to a gym and work out all day. He worked and waited for a reaction, observing and timing the symptoms and the recovery period. At the conclusion of his experiments he could read his diabetes as well as he could read opposing pitchers.

We wish we could give you a chart that would say something like, "For three sets of tennis take 20 ounces of orange juice," or "For eighteen holes of golf eat two scoops of ice cream." But it cannot be. The best we can do is give you a chart of calorie expenditures for various sports (see Appendix E). A chart like this, however, can only show you the relative degree of strenuousness of these sports. It can't show how much carbohydrate you as an individual will burn in a specific activity. Your metabolism, weight, the amount of vigor with which you play, and even the kind of weather you're playing in will determine how much food and insulin you need.

Either extremely hot or extremely cold weather makes the body work harder to maintain its thermostatic status quo, and if it's working harder it needs less insulin—or more food.

If you're a woman you have two more variables to consider: the menstrual cycle and pregnancy. One twenty-seven-year-old woman who is actively involved with skiing, biking, hiking, and tennis finds she gets more hypoglycemic attacks when her menstrual period is in progress.

A new mother reports, "I skied through my fifth month of pregnancy and my diabetes was more brittle [unstable] then. I was having insulin reactions more frequently and had to be extremely careful and certain to have plenty of sugar with me. If my husband and I went out dancing in the evening, I'd have to eliminate the injection of regular insulin I usually took before dinner when I was pregnant, and I'd also require a larger snack before I went to bed in order to avoid an insulin reaction during the night."

It's variables like these that make diabetes such a challenging game, and, like all games, the more you practice the better you get.

EITHER RAISE THE BRIDGE OR LOWER THE WATER

When you're exercising there are two main routes you can take to avoid the low-blood-sugar doldrums. You can eat quite a lot more or you can take less insulin and eat only a little more. By a ratio of about four to one, our contacts preferred the latter system.

"The amount of reduction depends upon the activity and the predicted work load. I may only reduce my normal 34 units by 4 units or may drop it to as low as one half normal for strenuous activities such as all-day backpacking."

"I usually lower my insulin about 4 units for field hockey and basketball, 2 units for softball and badminton."

"For skiing or bicycling all day, I cut my insulin by one third in the morning and one sixth at night, depending on how late exercise continues."

"Often I'll reduce by one third during an entire two- or three-week scuba-diving trip. Lately my doctor has suggested that . . . to drop to a low insulin intake for reasonable lengths of time is not a problem."

Dan Rowan lowers his insulin before playing in a tennis tournament. He doesn't want to have to eat any extra food because, unlike most insulin takers, he sometimes finds himself getting eight to ten pounds over his ideal weight.

Lowering the insulin dosage is definitely the better technique if for some reason you can't carry very much food—as in backpacking—or can't find the opportunity for snacking, as in scuba diving. Some sportspeople with extra high standards of cuisine mentioned that they preferred to lower their insulin dosage in order to avoid having to stuff down large quantities of poor-quality cafeteria food at ski resorts or other out-of-the-way places.

The eat-more-food advocates, though not in the majority, have some very explicit reasons for their point of

Shocking Experiences

view. Many of our diabetics are forbidden by their doctors to alter their insulin dosage on their own. For these people there is simply no alternative when exercising strenuously but to add calories and carbohydrates to the diet. Still others point out that their weight is more stable if they don't play with their insulin. They try never to change their insulin dosage except for an illness or infection.

Bill Talbert is one of those who prefer not to change the amount of insulin. Hockey pro Bobby Clarke is another. "I've tried to change insulin doses to help with control," Clarke says, "but I found it was easier for me to change my food intake to conform with my changing level of activity."

And then there are those who simply enjoy the extra food. "I am a foodaholic as well as a diabetic," says one, "so I certainly enjoy the snacks that are required because of excessive exercise."

Another agrees: "I am always starving when I ski and I don't even feel guilty about eating so much so often because I know I'm working it off as fast as I'm eating it."

It's the more professional, competitive athletes, however, who build the strongest case for the don't-tamper-with-your-insulin system. Professor Leete is one of these: "I have found that lowering my insulin also lowers my efficiency. I maintain the same dose of insulin and increase the food intake for prolonged effort."

The Maryland high school football linebacker mentioned earlier thinks that he plays much better and feels much better if he takes his full amount of insulin even though this means he must be extra careful about insulin reactions.

One seventeen-year-old bicycle racer has evolved a

unique method of handling insulin and food. The day before competing he *in*creases his injection slightly in order to be able to rest for twenty-four hours. Then, on the day of the race, he goes back to his regular insulin dosage and just before the start he eats a little more than usual.

A former program director at a diabetic camp in Ohio, and a diabetic himself, states: "Each three-week session we had a fifteen-mile hike for campers ages eleven through fifteen. We found that it was more effective to keep the same insulin dosage, but to allow the campers to eat all they wanted during the day of the hike. I feel a lot better doing it this way, too, especially the following day."

An additional point is that, if you rely on the extra food method instead of less insulin, you don't get in trouble if there is a change of plans and the sport session is canceled because of weather or one of the multitudinous common traffic or arrangement mishaps of modern life.

Some of the most active diabetic sportspeople neither lower their insulin nor raise their food, because they always keep up the same high daily pace of physical activity. As one of them—a horseman who competes in show jumping—tells it, "I try to remain as active physically as I can so that on the day of competition it's not that much more exercise than my actual training period."

An eighteen-year-old basketball and track star explains the one kind of insulin adjustment this system demands: "I *in*crease the dosage of insulin when I'm *not* going to be active. There aren't many days when I'm not working out."

One very athletic fourteen-year-old, whose specialty is wrestling, is what you might call ambi-insulinous. He

Shocking Experiences

goes both ways with his dosage. "It can be lowered up to five units on a day when I will be wrestling and raised up to five units on days when I will be sitting around."

As you can see, there's more than one way to inject a diabetic cat and still keep him on the fence between high and low blood sugar.

1+ TO GET READY

In order to avoid reactions in the middle of the action, some diabetics try for a slight spill as they start their sport. Bill Talbert, for instance, says, "I try to be slightly on the plus side and stay there during my exercise." A young wrestler agrees, saying that he holds off low blood sugar by "keeping Tes-Tape handy and my blood sugar a one plus when involved with a practice or a sports event." A football player tells us, "I feel that I play and feel much better with my sugar around one plus." One hiker resorts to "constant urine testing with the object of spilling small amounts most of the time, which helps to avoid most of the difficulty."

But what if you're not in a place where you can do the "constant urine testing," and what if you find it hard to spill exactly a trace or a one plus? On the theory that if a little is good more is better, how about giving yourself a big glucose insurance policy? Why not just always eat a lot of carbohydrate and make sure you're starting your activity with a good, healthy spill?

Well, in the first place, there's no such animal as a good, healthy spill. Spilling a lot of sugar is not good and not healthy. If you always start a sport with high blood sugar and you're a regular sports participant, it stands to reason you're going to be running—and swimming and skiing—around with high blood sugar a good part of the time.

Probably that wouldn't faze a fanatic athlete who wants to succeed at all physical costs: witness the athletes who wreck their health with drugs and steroids in order to flail a little more out of their bodies. A diabetic, though, can't trade giant spills for reaction elimination without risking something besides long-range health—namely, sports proficiency. Sports proficiency is decreased by high blood sugar to a considerable degree. For example, a tennis player reports, "Last summer in a tournament playoff I thought my blood sugar was low. I ate lots of carbohydrates. My blood sugar was high instead and I played miserably."

A bicyclist we talked to said he finds that, unless he anticipates a strenuous burst of energy at the beginning of a ride, it's much better for him not to eat too much, as this raises his blood sugar and makes his start sluggish.

So it seems that contrary to the philosopher Mae West —"Too much of a good thing can be wonderful"—when the good thing is a *slight* increase in blood sugar for a sport, too much of *that* good thing can be ruinous.

IT TAKES ONE TO KNOW ONE

Many diabetics have great confidence in their ability to read their bodies and especially to read their blood sugar. One twenty-three-year-old we talked to was into so many sports (karate, skiing, sailing, football, baseball, basketball, tennis, surfing, handball, motorcycles, and backpacking) that you'd think he wouldn't have a single waking minute available for monitoring his blood

Shocking Experiences

sugar. Still, he claims he can tell by the way he feels whether his sugar is high or low. You've got to believe him, because he has excellent control. On the last two visits to his doctor's office his sugar count was 75. Of course, this athlete does have a bit of experience with diabetes. He's twenty-three and has had it for twenty-one and a half years.

Some diabetics do not recognize a reaction coming on, and their shocks are fairly well developed before they or someone else realizes what is happening. The vast majority of diabetics, however, can identify their symptoms of low blood sugar most of the time—but, alas, not all the time. An example is Joe "Mr. Cincinnati" Brink, who says, "Usually I can feel myself getting low, but there are times that insulin reactions occurred and I didn't even feel myself going into them."

It's not surprising that low blood sugar is sometimes hard to recognize. The individual symptoms can vary tremendously:

"My whole personality changes and I become very belligerent and hard to reach."

"One night I woke up shaking and trembling. . . . I was seeing spots like mosquitoes all over the room."

"I've had insulin reactions while bowling. I would not be paying attention for my turn, and when it was my turn I'd bowl in the wrong alley, or try to bowl three times instead of the one or two times."

"My body feels light, my head is dizzy, and I feel weak. I start to shake, then fall into a deep sleep. It's a weirdout of a feeling."

"I was sweating and I couldn't keep my eyes open because I was too drowsy."

"In golf my shots aren't straight, or maybe I'm downright terrible for no apparent reason. Also, I sometimes see distant objects in double image."

In some cases it seems that coming out of a reaction can be as disquieting as going into one. Joe Brink reports that "at times I get belligerent when I start to come out of a reaction and start swinging my fists and seem to have extra strength and I'm sure this scares people sometimes."

Even the kind of insulin you take (regular, NPH, Lente, etc.) can influence the kind of reaction symptoms you get. If you change insulins, you need to alert yourself for possible new and strange low-blood-sugar sensations.

Besides this, we heard Dr. Russell Poucher, president of the American Diabetes Association, Southern California Affiliate, explain that the symptoms of reactions vary according to how fast your blood sugar is falling. If it's going down rapidly, you get the shakes, the sweats, the nasty disposition, the hunger, the palpitations, the nausea, and so on—in other words, the more dramatic and noticeable symptoms. You also get enlarged pupils, which is something you can alert your friends and family members to watch for.

When the blood sugar is dropping slowly but reaches the level at which the brain is deprived of its necessary glucose, you get the more cerebral symptoms, such as slurring of speech, blurring of vision, and confusion. If you get this kind of slowly lowering blood-sugar reaction in the night, it can cause nightmares and make you feel sluggish when you wake up in the morning.

Before June knew about these two distinct kinds of reactions she was never positive she was having a reaction when it was the slow, cerebral kind. She'd sit around wait-

Shocking Experiences

ing for something more definitive like the sweats to happen, all the time growing more and more vague and losing more and more of her reasoning powers. Thanks to Dr. Poucher's analysis, she can now recognize—and do something about—the more subtle cerebral symptoms.

TOUGHING IT OUT

What if you should start getting an insulin reaction at just the wrong time? (Is there ever a *right* time?) What if you're at game, set, and match point? What if you're in the middle of a hiking trail and you want to get to a cool shady waterfall picnic spot instead of the bug-infested swamp you've been slogging through? What if you're the quarterback and the score is 13–7 against your team and you're inside their 20-yard line and there's only time for about three more plays before the end-of-the-game gun goes off? These are the times when you'll want to grit your teeth and tighten up your stomach muscles and, with all the determination you can muster, hold onto your senses and motor control until a more convenient moment comes for downing your emergency carbohydrate ration. Yes, these are the times that try diabetics' souls. You *want* to hang in there, but, as a friend of ours likes to say, "People in hell want ice water." You have about as much chance of toughing out an insulin reaction as the hellions do of getting a refreshing drink.

Here is the diabetic voice of experience speaking on what to do when shock knocks:

"If the situation is one where I can get food, I eat immediately; otherwise I sit down and don't use unnecessary energy."

"I quit, rest, try to drink water if available, ask for some food, or proceed in a restful state to the nearest sources."

"Quit. If you don't, you'll learn the hard way."

In a competitive sports situation it's particularly important that you stop and do something at the first suspicion of an impending reaction. If you don't make your wise decision at the onset, it's likely to be too late in very short order. One of the first faculties to go is your decision-making ability. If you're on a team, the members will respect you much more if you have the sense to get out of the game and get yourself back together than if you try to hang in there and maybe blow it for everyone. When it comes to handling a reaction in sports, your brains—not your guts—are what are going to pull you out of it.

Still, some diabetic sportspeople think they can hold back the dawn of an insulin reaction. One skier we know of says, "I find if I concentrate on something in my mind I keep better control while the reaction is progressing. Thinking of a song or actually singing it keeps my mind sharp and lets me concentrate on control until I can get to food. As long as I can think of something, I feel I'm all right; and, for me, thinking does slow down the progress of a reaction."

Maybe this works for him, but frankly we'd hate to have anyone count on it. The only possible way singing *might* slow the progress of a reaction is if previously your activities were going to the beat of "Yankee Doodle" and you changed them to the rhythm of "Ol' Man River." The more slowly you move, the more slowly the reaction evolves. This is because our bodies consume fuel more or less as automobiles do. We all know from the lessons of the

Shocking Experiences

energy crisis that if we drive our Detroit gas guzzlers 55 mph we get more miles per gallon than if we drive them 75 mph; so, too, our internal glucose guzzlers. Cut your speed and you get more mileage out of the glucose that's still left in your tank.

It's an advantage, too, if you are one of those diabetics who are so familiar with their bodies that they know exactly how much time they have left before an incipient reaction becomes a fall-on-the-floor affair. Lead times vary dramatically from five or ten minutes to as long as an hour. One skier even admitted, "If I am skiing down the slope and I feel an insulin reaction coming, I don't run to the lodge and eat. I take two or three more runs—slower, of course—then I go in. I don't think every diabetic can do this, but I feel I can because I know my body so well."

But just to keep you on the straight and narrow, we'll also give you the far, far more typical and recommended approach. "At first sign of shock, the very first sign, I start looking for a source of food. I usually have about ten to fifteen minutes before I really get into a spot. So far I haven't gotten into any, but I don't feel that it can't happen to me."

SUMMERTIME, WHEN THE SHOCKING IS EASY

We mentioned before that a change in the weather can change your insulin requirement. The body has to work to maintain its temperature when the outside temperature is lower or higher than the normal 98.6 degrees. As we know, work burns up blood sugar and lowers your insulin need (or increases your food need).

It would logically seem that more shocks would occur

in winter, when the outside temperature is around 32 degrees, than in summer, when it might be in the 90- to 100-degree range. In winter the temperature is farther from the body's normal level. Logic doesn't seem to work in this case, though. Almost all the temperature-induced insulin reactions that were reported to us took place in hot weather.

A Canadian diabetic experienced the only reaction of his life that took him to the point of unconsciousness as a result of going to warm Florida from the frozen North, but at least he learned from the experience. "I've been to Florida a number of times since then," he says. "I drop my insulin as I enter into a warmer climate, and I've not had any trouble with the diabetes in connection with being in a warmer climate since."

The Maryland linebacker has also had a mighty reaction experience in hot weather. "Once during the two-a-day football practice this past fall I really had about the worst one that I have experienced since becoming a diabetic. It was an unusually hot day, around 95 degrees, and I hadn't eaten much lunch between the practices. I got shaky and felt as though I was going to pass out but orange juice brought me around."

Even Ron Santo, when he was playing third base for the Chicago Cubs, occasionally had temperature-induced problems.

"It seemed like a cool day in Chicago. I took a little extra insulin before the game. But it turned out to be a hot day. By the ninth inning, I was getting dizzy. There was a man on first and one on second and I was at bat. I didn't want to cop out, but I was hoping I would strike out, so I could get back to the bench and eat the candy bar the

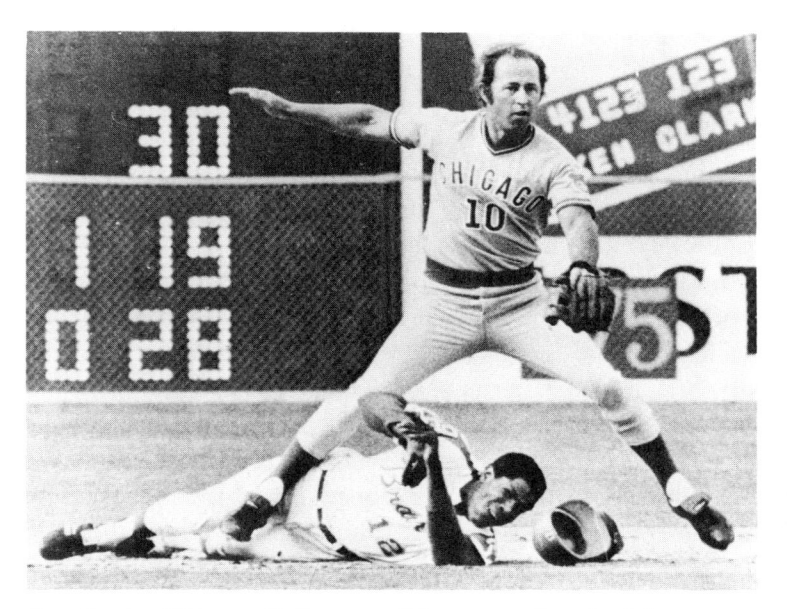

Ron Santo, Chicago Cubs second baseman, knocked the word "handicap" out of the ballpark. (UPI Photo)

trainer always keeps for me." As luck would have it, Santo hit a home run and had to run around the bases to make it to the candy.

It isn't always the weather that heats you up and throws off your insulin requirement. Clothing can do it, too—at least, somewhat unusual clothing can. An eighteen-year-old Californian named Theresa Harris—scuba diver, water skier, and motorcycle rider—is a very active member of Fire Explorer Scouts. (The Boy Scouts is no longer a sexist organization!) As part of a fund-raising promotion for that group Theresa is sometimes called upon to put on a heavy Smokey the Bear suit—including the furry head cover—and ride on a fire engine or trot about shopping malls. "Twice around the mall," states Theresa, "and it's reaction time."

Possibly hot weather affects insulin needs more than cold, because it's easier to keep your body warm in winter clothes than it is to keep it cool in summer clothes. After all, you can add clothing almost indefinitely, but there's a point beyond which you cannot go in taking it off. Even at a nudist colony, if the temperature's over a hundred, the body's going to have to work to cool itself. (Unfortunately we've had no dealings with diabetic nudists, so we can't give a personal experience statement on this.)

Dr. Olson has come up with another sound speculation about why more shocks seem to happen in hot rather than in cold weather. "With the advent of warmer weather in the spring, most of us are more active physically, and even a sixty-year-old fat diabetic who does not ordinarily get much exercise may decide to walk to the store instead of jumping into the car and riding there. The additional amount of exercise certainly has some effect on insulin requirements."

WHEN IS A REACTION NOT A REACTION?

One controversy we've come across has to do with the effect of fear on blood-sugar levels. Say you're about to ski off a cornice or hang-glide off a cliff and you're scared witless and spitless—so scared that your body starts squirting out adrenaline. Does this cause hypoglycemia or hyperglycemia? Our high-risk sports-minded diabetics reported mainly that this kind of physical terror gives them low blood sugar. But is this true?

It certainly is true that an adrenaline hype *feels* exactly like insulin shock. But according to our expert, Dr. Olson, what is going on inside your body is the opposite of

Shocking Experiences

what you think. Adrenaline is an insulin antagonist. This means that it blocks the action of insulin and triggers the release of glucose from the liver, causing the blood sugar to go up.

This is quite logical if you stop to think about it. In a state of fear the body tries to marshal all its resources to prepare for facing a threat—the old "fight or flight" reaction. A good supply of the energy fuel, glucose, does indeed give you the basic resource for fast escape or standing and fighting off the challenge. This sudden excessive supply of adrenaline in the system causes sweating, shakiness, and excessive hunger, the same cues you get when you're going into the first stages of insulin shock. The body sensations are identical for insulin or adrenaline shock. The body reacts to fear in the same way it reacts to dangerously falling blood sugar: it secretes adrenaline. (In fact, just to further complicate matters, an insulin reaction caused by rapidly falling blood sugar is sometimes called an "adrenaline-type reaction.")

These warning signals—sweating, shakiness, and excessive hunger—are so familiar to you as insulin-shock symptoms that you interpret them as such. In a fear situation, though, what you probably have is adrenaline shock, which will proceed to deliver glucose to your bloodstream on top of whatever sugar is already there, even if it's normal or on the high side. If you eat to counteract the false low-blood-sugar symptoms, you can see what galloping high blood sugar you can make for yourself.

Fortunately, when you're in one of these extreme fear situations you probably won't have an opportunity to eat. As one diabetic says, "In skydiving it's a little hard to stop for a candy bar on the way down."

Of course, there is the possibility that you could, as in the case of skiing a new steep and difficult run, have low blood sugar and fear hit you at the same time. In this case, your liver delivery of glucose might not be sufficient to bring you up again without extra food. It's obviously not easy to analyze and take care of.

If you don't make it a habit to scare yourself out of your mind every day, it probably wouldn't hurt in this confusing—and confused—state to chomp down some Life Savers or, as one salty-talking sugar eater puts it, "hit the cubes." As you know, most doctors advise that when in doubt you should treat for low blood sugar. Just don't be mystified if you wind up spilling like crazy.

SHOCK BUSTERS

When it comes to reaction counteractors, a diabetic needs two kinds: one kind for emergencies to be used when you're really into a reaction and another kind for when you're just experiencing hints and mild harbingers of low blood sugar and you want to both counteract that and give yourself a little long-range buildup to prevent future problems. We'll discuss the latter in the section on snacks. Right now, emergency rations are on the bill of fare.

Glucagon. In the greatest of emergencies—that is, when you're unconscious—an injection of glucagon is the best and fastest and safest (no choking possibility) way out. Glucagon can be injected in exactly the same way as insulin.

Contrary to what you may think from its name, glucagon is not a sugar (like glucose) but rather a hormone, like insulin. This hormone is produced by the alpha cells of the pancreas just as insulin is produced by the beta cells. Glucagon works in the opposite way from insulin. Insulin lowers the blood sugar; glucagon raises it. The way it does this is to stimulate the liver to convert its glycogen supply into glucose. As a matter of fact, it is now believed that diabetes is not just a problem of underproduction of insulin but one of overproduction of glucagon as well. Doctors call it "a bihormonal disease."

The obvious flaw with using glucagon is that if you're unconscious you can't give it to yourself, and the average person who comes upon your inert form isn't going to be able to rummage through your knapsack, find the glucagon, read the instructions, mix it up, and inject it. So really glucagon is only of use if you have a family member or friend or coach who can administer it.

There is an enthusiastic skier in British Columbia who keeps the ski patrol supplied with glucagon because "when severe insulin shock . . . does occur usually I'm not aware of the symptoms; consequently I just crash. . . . The guys just check for breathing, heart rate, keep me warm, mix and inject glucagon I.M. into the hip area, and transport me to the First Aid hut where, by then, they can feed me orange juice and other carbohydrates to keep the blood sugar up there until control is reestablished. . . . We find glucagon works really well in these situations and consciousness usually returns in ten to fifteen minutes."

The only other method we've heard of that is a safe and effective way to bring around a totally unconscious diabetic is an enema of Karo syrup, Coke syrup, or honey—and most people would prefer administering glucagon to that.

Instant Glucose. This form of glucose is as fast-acting as anything else you can take orally. Since it's already in a semiliquid state, the body doesn't have to do any further work on it to make it assimilable. An additional advantage is that it can be administered to you by an informed companion if you're too far gone to handle the situation yourself. (He smears a little on the inside of your cheek; you won't choke on it the way you would on a liquid.)

Instant glucose is also handy to carry, because it comes in a tube. Nothing's perfect, though. Thom Underwood, of Bend, Oregon, whom we think of as "the hip shooter" because of his with-it way of talking about and handling his diabetes, says of instant glucose, "Used to carry those tubes of glucose but they burst and they're filthy buggers to have in a coat. Too damn sticky."

Another problem with instant glucose is that, sweet as it may be, yummy it is not. June used to carry it, but she never used it to any great extent. In the first place, she never let herself get into a real emergency situation, and for a semiemergency she never wanted to "eat that sickening guck." On the one occasion she had any contact with it, she touched her finger to the instant glucose and then to the tip of her tongue the way movie detectives taste a substance to see if it has poison in it. At least with instant glucose, though, you don't ever snack on it for pleasure when it's not really needed.

Instant glucose can be ordered from:

> The Diabetes Association of Greater Cleveland
> 2022 Lee Road
> Cleveland, Ohio   44118

As we write this, the cost is $2 for three tubes.

Reactose. Up in Dr. Olson's bailiwick, the Deaconess Hospital in Spokane, the popular favorite form of fast glucose is Reactose. This is in a more liquid form than instant glucose; consequently, it comes in a plastic bottle instead of a tube. Each two-ounce bottle contains 32 grams of glucose and is equipped with a twist-and-squirt top which has an unfortunate tendency to get gummed up. The directions and bottle markings, however, are very clear and explicit. Anyone with a sixth-grade reading ability could figure out quickly how to administer it in a pinch.

Dr. Olson considers Reactose more convenient to carry and easier to use than its stickier cousin. June considers it slightly less sickening in taste, although it does smack of lemon-flavored castor oil.

Reactose can be ordered from:

> C. R. Canfield & Company
> 2744-46 Lyndale Avenue South
> Minneapolis, Minnesota 55408

The cost is $2.25 for a two-ounce bottle.

Dextrose Cubes. Dextrose is a form of glucose, and these cubes are often imported, usually expensive, but always handy, since they dissolve and take effect very quickly. These are available in most hiking and camping stores.

EASY RISERS

Moving right along in the lineup of blood-sugar raisers, we come to several others that are more common products and, hence, more readily obtainable.

Honey. Honey is very good since it's a liquid, it's concentrated, and half of its sugar is glucose. That rascal, Colonel

Sanders, has stopped giving out those handy packs of honey with his chicken dinners unless you specifically ask for them—as of course you should, because they're diabetically very useful.

Fruit Juices. Fruit juices are popular because of their good taste and availability. They also have the advantage of containing vitamins. Grape juice, because it's about half glucose, is the fastest acting, but orange juice is the favorite choice.

We have heard of a double dose of blood-sugar raiser, used by people who really wanted to blast themselves out of a reaction: They pour sugar into a glass of orange juice and gulp it all down. Beware! This combination can backfire on you—literally. Dr. Russell Poucher explains that sugar plus orange juice may be just too much to handle. It can cause a spasm resulting in vomiting up the whole concoction.

A combination of honey and orange juice apparently doesn't have the same disastrous effect, at least not for everyone. One skier takes this double whammy of a blood-sugar raiser along in a bota bag. Not only does this keep the mix handy, it makes him look like a real swinger on the slopes.

Other diabetics report carrying orange juice in canteens when they're on hikes. Some substitute that wine of outer space, Tang, which they say works as well as the real stuff. One guy, to save space, just uses Tang in its crystal form.

Soft Drinks. Dr. Poucher's recommendation for the best reaction fighter is a soft drink. He's found 7-Up to be particularly good, but any soft drink—Coke, root beer, ginger

Shocking Experiences

ale, Orange Crush, Dr. Pepper, to name a few—is fine. The advantage of soft drinks is that they are usually easy to get; soft-drink machines abound in so-called civilized areas. The disadvantages of soft drinks are: (1) you have to have change available to use a soft-drink machine; (2) when you're in a noncivilized area these machines *don't* abound, and cans and bottles of soft drinks are very heavy and cumbersome to tote; (3) in this weight-conscious modern world more and more often soft drinks are sugar free or virtually sugar free. Sometimes, in a punchy state, the diabetic is not able to recognize the difference, and sometimes well-meaning friends who go to fetch the soft drink for the in-reaction diabetic deliberately get the sugar-free variety, because they can't get it through their heads that a diabetic sometimes desperately *needs* sugar.

Sugar. This old standby works faster if it's dissolved in water but is usually fast enough for most purposes when eaten as is. A skier reports, "One time in Steamboat Springs, Colorado, I had to run into a town restaurant and pour sugar from a table container into my hand and lick it down." Rather than resort to this, however, most diabetics prefer to carry those little packets of "that terrible granulated sugar," as one of them calls it, for an emergency. Better still are what Thom Underwood calls "the cubes." He's discovered two good carrying containers: boxes for Band-Aids or Sucrets (those foil-wrapped throat lozenges).

Life Savers. Life Savers are very handy and very fast-acting—faster than sugar actually, because they contain corn syrup, a form of glucose. They also taste good. As a result they are very popular with diabetics. Some prefer Charms because they are individually wrapped, but they're not as easy to find in stores.

Chocolate Candy. Bars of this tasty substance are more popular than they should be. They *will* raise your blood sugar, but not as fast as other candies because many chocolate bars contain more fat than sugar.

FIRST ADE?

Several diabetics we talked to wondered whether or not those special sports drinks like Gatorade, E.R.G., and Sportade might be good to bring a diabetic out of hypoglycemia. (After all, according to their ads, they are good for whatever else might ail a sportsperson.) We wondered about them, too, so we asked Dr. Olson about them.

Dr. Olson had thoroughly investigated these electrolyte-replacement drinks when he was writing his book, *Prevention of Football Injuries.* He concluded that using any of the "ades" in treating hypoglycemic reactions would be objectionable from two standpoints: "(1) their cost and (2) the fact that they contain sodium and potassium in addition to the sugar. Certain diabetics should not be taking in extra sodium, and most of them do not have any need for extra potassium. It is much cheaper to simply stir up 2 teaspoons of sugar in a glass of water, and it is really just as effective. Sportade has about 12 grams of sugar per 8-ounce glass and it is mostly sucrose (table sugar). Gatorade is all glucose and has essentially around 12.5 grams in an 8-ounce glass, but a tablespoon of Karo would give you a little more than that and is less volume and easier to get down at once. Halftime Punch is all sucrose and again is no better than table sugar stirred in a glass of water."

HOW MUCH, HOW FAST?

It is impossible to say exactly how much of your chosen blood-sugar raiser it will take to pull you out of a reaction. It depends on all kinds of personal, physical, and activity factors. Still, there are some guidelines. At the Diabetes Education Center at the Deaconess Hospital in Spokane, patients are given a copy of this sugar content chart of suggested foods for reactions.

Corn syrup (Karo)	1 tbsp. = 15 grams
Honey	1 tbsp. = 16 grams
Maple syrup	1 tbsp. = 13 grams
Life Savers	3 candies = 10 grams
Cube sugar	2 cubes = 12 grams
Packet of sugar (1 level tsp.)	2 packets = 8 grams
Orange juice	½ cup = 10 grams
Sweetened soda pop	½ cup = 20 grams
Jam	1 rounded tsp. = 14 grams
Jelly	1 rounded tsp. = 13 grams

Dr. Olson, the Center's director, explains that anything which is the equivalent of 10 to 15 grams of glucose will usually bring the average diabetic out of a reaction, but occasionally you may need to double the amount.

The Joslin Clinic in its *Diabetes Teaching Guide* offers similar advice: "TREAT ALL REACTIONS IMMEDIATELY. Take a simple fast-acting sugar and allow it 10 to 15 minutes to act. Repeat the same dose of sugar if no improvement with the first."

But, when you come right down to it, getting exactly the right amount of sugar for a reaction is generally not something you have to get uptight about. As Dr. Olson points out, "Actually we just advise all our diabetics to carry a couple of rolls of Life Savers or half a dozen sugar cubes, and in most instances this does the trick nicely."

OVERKILL

Dave Engerbretson has described a scenario almost all insulin-taking diabetics have been through in a reaction.

"The feeling of hunger is so overpowering that I feel I just can't get enough in there fast enough and generally I overdo it. I eat so much junk that the blood sugar bounces back the other way and then I've got a headache and I'm sick to my stomach and got to have an Alka-Seltzer and I feel terrible.

"If I had enough sense to eat what I know is going to do the job and then just go and lie down and wait for it to hit me, I would be better. Instead, I seem to keep eating until the feeling goes away and by that time I've way overdone it. But then, when there's a nice chocolate cake sitting there, things you don't normally eat, it's kind of nice to overdo it."

It takes more than just "enough sense" not to overkill a reaction. It takes an almost uncanny ability to figure out exactly what the right amount is, and it takes a huge amount of self-control in the face of either a raging hunger such as the one Dave describes or, even more common, a terrible fear that you're heading into a deep reaction and you'd better get out of it as fast as possible. You keep eating until the symptoms leave. Then by the time they do leave, of course, you're stuck with sky-high blood sugar.

Shocking Experiences

This kind of anxiety eating sometimes takes place when your blood sugar isn't even low, but when you just *think* it is—or should be. After exercising June has sometimes stuffed a lot of food down, only to find at her next urine test that her symptoms weren't low blood sugar at all but merely ordinary fatigue.

We wish there were a magic formula to give you to avoid blood-sugar overkill, but all we have to offer are Dextrostix (explained in the following section). Should you find with a Dextrostix that your symptoms are for real, then use a big helping of self-control along with the blood-sugar-raising food. Try to eat what *you've* learned from experience is enough to bring *you* back to normal. (June has ascertained that it takes 20 grams of carbohydrate—for example, 8 ounces of orange juice or 4 lumps of sugar—to raise her blood-glucose level from 40 to 120.) After eating, stop and rest and wait for the food to take effect. Wait at least fifteen minutes. Try to relax and don't whip yourself into an emotional frenzy that will produce false low-blood-sugar symptoms. And, above all, don't use your real or imagined low blood sugar as an excuse to overdo on something like Dave's chocolate cake!

A STIX IN TIME

One situation it's smart to avoid is beginning a sports activity with low blood sugar. You're likely to have a reaction before you even get out of the starting gate. But how are you going to know if your blood sugar is low? A handy-dandy urine test—or even an unhandy-undandy one—only tells you if you're spilling. If you're not spilling, you could be in the normal range or a little low or so low as to be on the brink of a reaction. There's no way, with a urine test, to differentiate.

Not only that, but even if you *are* spilling you could still be low. Your urine test could be reflecting a spill of an hour ago, if you haven't done what is called a "second void." That is, you urinate once to get rid of past history and then you do it again half an hour later so that your test reports what's going on in the body fairly close to the present. (Even a half hour later, though, if your blood sugar is dropping rapidly a second void may be deceptive.)

Fortunately, there is a way other than urine tests to get a reading of your blood sugar, and this is a much more valid one. You use Dextrostix, made by the Ames Company. This product, which measures blood sugar from a finger prick, isn't widely advertised and not everyone has heard of it. Out of the over 150 diabetics we worked with, only three mentioned using it. We ourselves were aware of its existence but were unclear about what it did and how it did it.

The first specific recommendation of Dextrostix we ever read was in an article on travel for diabetics written by Dr. Stanley Mirsky in *Diabetes Forecast*. Dr. Mirsky advised that the diabetic's traveling companions carry the "stix" so that in case the diabetic was ever found unconscious they would be prepared to determine quickly whether the cause was hypoglycemia or hyperglycemia (insulin shock or diabetic coma).

Hmm, we thought, these Dextrostix might be just the thing for seeing where you stand before you leap into a sports activity. We set out to find some to experiment with. After checking with several pharmacies, June finally had

Shocking Experiences

to special-order them. Pharmacists, at least in our area, not only didn't regularly stock Dextrostix but many seemed quite vague as to what they were. They are, we found, little plastic sticks about three inches long with (to use pharmaceutical talk) an "impregnated reagent area affixed," like Ketostix, another Ames product you may be familiar with. What Dextrostix do is give you an instant—well, actually it takes about three minutes——blood-sugar reading.

All you do is prick your finger and get a big drop of blood. For this June uses an old disposable insulin injection needle and syringe, although you can buy special lances. You put the blob of blood on the reagent area, time it for exactly sixty seconds, and wash it off with water for one or two seconds. Then you compare the reagent area with the color chart on the side of the Dextrostix bottle.

The color chart has seven gradations of color indicating blood-sugar levels of 0, 25, 45, 90, 130, 175, and 250 or more. You have to guess for blood-sugar scores in between, but you have to do a lot of guessing anyway, because it's very difficult to match the sticks accurately with the color chart unless you are blessed with superb color acuity. June found it easy, though, to decide whether her blood sugar was extremely low or extremely high, and she decided the best use of Dextrostix was to determine if you were either bordering on or deeply into hypoglycemia. Since that's precisely how a sportsperson will be using them, they are ideal either before or after great energy expenditures.

What are the drawbacks of Dextrostix? Well, folks, these mini-magic wands ain't cheap. If you buy them by the hundred, they cost about 43 cents each. In the twenty-five-stick container, they come to 50 cents apiece. But June is now hooked on them. In fact, she uses them not just in conjunction with sports but at those times when she has confusing body signals and can't sort out whether they're telling her her blood sugar is very low or very high.

If you are a superaffluent person and want to spend even more, say about $350, you can take all the guesswork out of using Dextrostix by also purchasing an Ames Eyetone Reflectance Colorimeter. You insert the Dextrostix into this little machine after you've washed off the blood, and it registers your exact blood sugar from 10 to 400. We think the meter would be especially useful for professional athletes in competition or for someone who is a brittle diabetic living in a wilderness area far from doctors and hospitals.

Although you don't need a prescription for Dextrostix, you can't get the meter without a doctor's prescription. If you have the tenacity of a terrier and the patience of Job, as well as a cooperative doctor, you may be able to persuade your health insurance to pay as much as 80 percent of the cost of the Colorimeter.

URINE BUSINESS

Although our friend Dick Bernstein was the first patient in the United States to own a Colorimeter and he now has two—one at home and one at the office—he realizes that you can't always have your meter with you. You may not even always have your Diastix or Tes-Tape with you. But Dick still has a way for you to test your urine.

Shocking Experiences

It involves no special equipment or materials whatsoever. It's a taste test. Yep, just as the doctors of ancient Greece and Rome tasted their patients' urine to see if it was sweet, you can do the same to see if you're spilling sugar. Even a trace of sugar will be detectable. Dick assures us that you don't have to worry about tasting being unsanitary, because urine is sterile.

Just to be sure about this, we checked with a learned microbiologist at the college where we work. She confirmed that, yes, urine is sterile when it leaves the bladder —but when it leaves the body it picks up bacteria from the skin. Even then, however, it has no more bacteria than, say, the average drinking water you're likely to come across.

Dick adds one caution. Artificial sweeteners can be tasted in the urine, so if you've been eating or drinking products that have been artificially sweetened your taste test will be inaccurate. Thus we conclude the description of what we think is the suggestion in this book least likely to be tried by our readers.

3

Preparations and Precautions

We've heard repeatedly from active sports-minded diabetics that diabetics can do anything other people can, if they just mind their P's and Q's or, rather, their P's and P's—preparations and precautions. With these two as basic sports equipment, diabetics can prevent most emergencies and cope with the few that manage to get through their lines of defense.

The best thing about a conscientious preparation and precaution program, though, is that it leaves your mind free during the activity for the challenge and fun of simply Doing It. Your mind is not unnecessarily preoccupied with diabetes.

SHOW AND TELL

A prime precaution for all diabetics is to tell their friends about their diabetes and to explain to them what can be done in an emergency. When it comes to this basic preventive strategy, though, not all diabetics have managed to work it out. Some do the wrong thing for the wrong reason, some do the wrong thing for the right reason, and some do the right thing for the wrong reason.

The-wrong-thing-for-the-wrong-reason doers are the worst off. They're the closet diabetics. They don't tell people about their disease, because they're embarrassed or ashamed or afraid people won't like them because of it.

Thom Underwood has a few words to set this group straight. "Don't be a fool and hide it. I would like to know what it is that shames you. You got it—so what? Ask yourself who makes you fearful to say, I am a diabetic! . . . Let people in your sport know; don't surprise them with insulin shock and make them dance and worry. Let 'em know. They'll watch you." When we asked Thom about how other people felt when he let them know he had diabetes, he said, "The ones that mattered didn't think anything about it."

And we particularly like a New Jersey football player's approach toward his teammates. "They don't feel too bad about it or make jokes about it, because when I play football, I am an animal, and they know that I'll break their heads. Plus, I think they respect me because I have diabetes and have accepted it."

Then there are those who do the wrong thing for the right reason or, at least, a more justifiable reason than some. They don't tell because they don't want to be a bother or to create a scene about the disease and send people into a flap. A Montana skier and backpacker has told us he is particularly bugged by people who "make a big fuss over you. . . . I found very few so-called mature adults who could handle the situation without making some kind of fuss. In other words, they made it worse."

Admittedly, these flappers can drive you nuts over the slightest diabetic problem, but mercifully they get over it in time when they finally realize the magic a little carbohydrate can work. You certainly shouldn't jeopardize your safety because of a few people who are by nature the kind that get hysterical over the slightest of life's irregularities. Just figure that, if they weren't flapping over you, they'd be flapping over someone or something else. You're probably performing a public service by getting someone else off the fusser's hook.

The idea that you don't tell because you don't want to be a bother to your friends or create a scene can backfire. Suppose your friends don't know you're a diabetic and you do go into insulin shock; they may think, if you get irritable and mean, that you hate them for no good reason, which is hardly a way to make them feel happy. If you grow vague and irrational, they may think that you're losing your mind—not a pleasant and undisturbing situation. If you go all the way and pass out, who knows what they'll think is wrong with you? Whatever they think, they're probably not going to be calm about it.

Most straight-thinking diabetics believe others should know about their diabetes in order to avoid embarrassment, both yours and theirs, during insulin reactions —to say nothing of how they'd feel if their ignorance should somehow cost you your life!

Ron Santo had his own kind of right reason for doing the wrong thing. He kept his diabetes hidden from his Chicago Cubs teammates for five years and from the general public for even longer. He did this because he didn't want people to feel sorry for him or say his diabetes was to blame when things weren't going well for him in a game.

Then there's doing the right thing—telling about your diabetes—for the wrong reason. What could a wrong reason be? It's fear. One sportswoman we know of, a gymnastics enthusiast, has this to say:

Preparations and Precautions 93

"To me one of the most heartbreaking things I've noted about diabetics met in classrooms, the gym, on trips, is the fear which shows itself with a very early statement of their diabetic condition. . . . I talk about being a diabetic when it is topical or natural in the conversation, but I do not *any longer* (I knew that fear firsthand) have the compulsion to let the crowd know I am worrying about the possibility of an emergency."

Now at last we arrive at doing the right thing for the right reason. Actually, there are two good right reasons, a selfish one and an altruistic one. The selfish reason for telling friends and teammates is that their knowledge of your condition and what to do about it may save your diabetic bacon. After all, should you turn non compos mentis or even totally unconscious, who is going to take the action to get you right again, if no one knows what's wrong and how to handle the situation? Where, for example, would one of our diabetic sportsmen have been in this situation without his informed friends?

"Walking to class I felt dizzy and the next thing I knew I woke up in the hospital. Friends told me later that I had staggered, fallen to the ground, and then started mildly convulsing. Thanks to their knowledge of my condition, they acted immediately and got me to the hospital and I.V. glucose."

And what would have happened to another diabetic when he charged out the door without his candy? "A few times kids have had to run around the ski hill finding sugar for Eric. . . . He forgot to take his candy with him. Everyone knows he has diabetes and therefore people will help him if he needs it."

It's not just in emergency situations that you need friends who know the diabetic score. As the aforementioned self-styled "animal" football player in New Jersey says of his best friend, football buddy, and roommate, "He has helped me out an awful lot. When I got down, he picked me up. He has given me my shots at times when I needed help. It's wonderful to have a friend like that and I love him for it." Letting your friends help you with your problems and returning the favor when they need it is what makes friends friends instead of just people who chug past each other in life on separate tracks.

The altruistic right reason for telling about your diabetes and how to handle it is that you're not just telling for one person's benefit but for the benefit of over ten million people in this country alone. You're spreading information that will help all Diabeteskind.

This was the right reason that caused Ron Santo in August 1971 to finally tell the world about his diabetes. He wanted to help other diabetics, especially children, to "learn to swing the bat and be independent." His official coming-out party was at a Diabetes Association of Greater Chicago Summer Camp for Diabetic Children, where he spoke to a group of a hundred. The members of the press, who had been keeping Ron's secret, were told that now they could reveal it.

But you don't have to be famous to do the right thing for the right reason. If every diabetic spoke out openly about this condition, diabetes knowledge would be as common as, say, the details of popular movie stars' romantic entanglements.

Sometimes it's not even a question of explaining to one's friends. One skier and businessman tells us that he actually relies on strangers. "My ski trips are usually in conjunction with business trips and I usually travel alone.

I try to stay at lodges that have dormitory accommodations. This makes it easier to meet people, and when I explain my condition they are most understanding. They can also get help if I should have a bad reaction. So far, this has never happened, but I feel better staying in a room with other people who are aware of my condition. The insulin shot first thing in the morning makes it easy to discuss my diabetes, and most people are very interested and ask many questions."

One caution here, though, is that when you do tell you must explain well and thoroughly about diabetes and what to do for shock and why. Semi-informed people are worse than no help at all. They know diabetics aren't supposed to eat sugar, so when you need some form of sugar for a reaction they are reluctant to help you get it. A little diabetic learning is a dangerous thing. So when you tell, tell all.

PLAYING SOLITAIRE

There are many great and good reasons why a diabetic shouldn't exercise alone. One of the best is that the sport may be one that nobody, whether diabetic or not, should do alone. As a Colorado sportsman puts it, "Normally, hunting or skiing should not be done alone by anyone, for if you should be off trail or off a run or a long way from camp or civilization, whether skiing or hunting, and break a leg, you will have a problem." Swimming or horseback riding by yourself are also risky—for nondiabetics as well as for diabetics.

But the hazards a diabetic faces in such don't-do-it-alone sports are, as always, even greater than the nondiabetic's risks. A diabetic has to consider not only the possibility of "normal" accidents like broken legs and swimming emergencies but insulin reactions as well. Joe Brink is adamant about not doing weight lifting alone, because he believes any weight lifter should have what they call a spotter. This is usually another person who is working out at the same time. If the weight lifter tries to lift a weight that's too heavy, the spotter can come to the rescue. Joe feels—and rightly so—that being a diabetic makes it even more important to work out with someone else, someone who understands insulin reactions in case anything should happen. He makes it a strict personal rule never to work out alone, nor does he let anyone at his gym do so.

Since we're trying to tell it as it is and not just as it should be under ideal conditions, we admit that, while some diabetics have sports companions all the time, some only have companions some of the time. For example, one horse trainer and horsewoman we know of only feels she needs to have someone around when she's working a young horse under saddle for the first few times.

Although Dick Bernstein enjoyed his weight lifting more when he worked out with friends in a health club near his office, he now exercises alone in the gym he built at home. He's really not running a horrendous risk by exercising alone, as he's not far from family help should he need it. Besides, he always works out right after dinner, when reaction risks are minimal. He doesn't need a spotter, either, because he's equipped his gym with a Universal Weight Lifting Machine, which automatically prevents possible injury. But the price of weight-lifting safety in solitude comes high. Those machines cost a hefty $3,000.

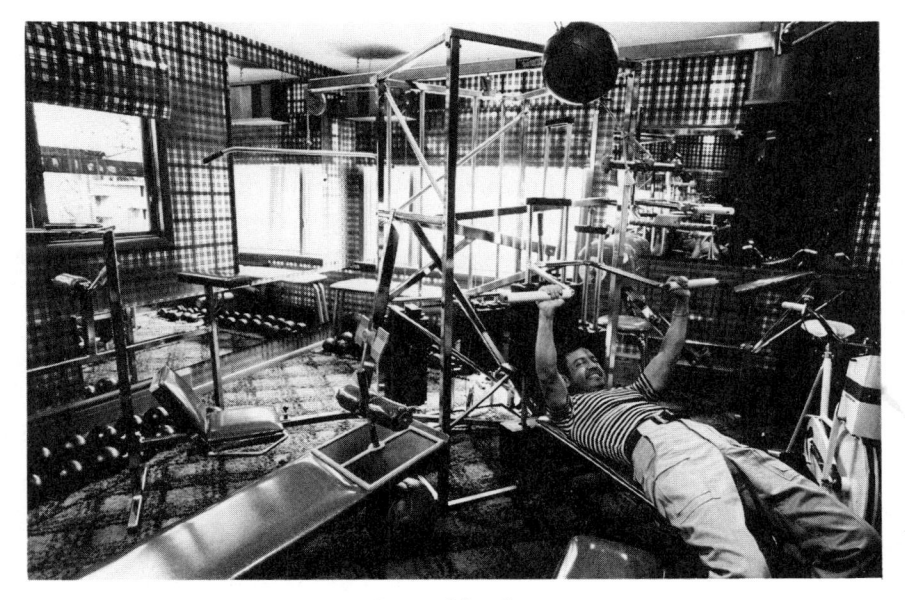

Weight lifter Dick Bernstein showed his heavy commitment to his exercise program by building this gym in his home.

We found that, of all the sports, running and jogging were the ones most often done alone.

"The only sport I practice alone is jogging. Since I've only jogged about two and a half miles at one time, it hasn't caused me any problems. It is quite vigorous while I'm jogging but it lasts only a short time—ten minutes at the most, so that doesn't give me too much of a chance to develop a severe insulin reaction."

Then there are the basic loners who find companions more of a problem than an aid and comfort:

"I prefer to do my sports alone. When I pack I have only once had anybody with me. I also enjoy sailing by myself more than having a bunch of people who don't know the difference between a jib and a mainsheet."

"Backpacking and bicycling trips by myself have presented no problems."

"I'm careful when I'm by myself, and also can pace myself and do not have to keep up with anyone else or conform to their appetites, so that I can eat when I think I need to and as a result I think I have less trouble when I'm alone."

If they're exercising for the sake of exercise and not as a pleasurable activity, some people find they get through more quickly if they work out alone. For example, Dick Bernstein says his weight-lifting routine takes one hour when he does it alone, but when his kids work out with him it takes two hours.

Some diabetics do things alone, but they admit they know they shouldn't. Dave Engerbretson is a member of the 4,000-footer club of New England. This means he's climbed all forty-six of the over 4,000-foot mountains in that area. "I don't remember if I climbed thirteen of them alone or all but thirteen of them alone, but at any rate I climbed an awful lot of them alone and that was pretty stupid. I think that most of the time a diabetic shouldn't be out there alone, no matter how well he understands the disease. You could . . . get into some severe problems that aren't even related to the diabetes."

A New England backpacker also takes a few guilt feelings along with her extra food and clothing when she hikes by herself. "In recent years I have received more than one lecture on the folly of hiking alone from people I've met on the trail (propaganda from the Forest Service, Appalachian Mountain Club, etc., seems to be taking hold). In attempting to persuade these nervous gentlemen that I am not totally rash and inexperienced, I fear that I have neglected to mention that I am a diabetic, lest they fly to the nearest Fish and Game warden (who

Preparations and Precautions

are in charge of rescue activities in the White Mountains)."

All diabetics agree, however, that if you do exercise alone you have to understand your disease thoroughly and redouble your already doubled precautions:

"If I practice alone I don't overplay, never have any problems. Anyway, I never go anywhere without sufficient fruit."

"When I'm alone I know I can't depend on anyone else, so if I start feeling funny I immediately rest and I also carry food and sugar with me at all times."

A young Massachusetts skier, cyclist, and swimmer made a particularly important point when she said, "I did find when I first got out of the hospital after my diagnosis of diabetes that I had to cut back on insulin and did go into many shocks. At this point, before being stabilized, there was a fear of being alone because I was just getting to understand diabetes and the various symptoms of insulin reaction. Also, before being completely stabilized, it was dangerous to participate in sports alone." In her opinion, "Once being stabilized and knowing what to expect, there is no reason for fear."

Kipling's line about "He travels fastest who travels alone" may apply to a diabetic sportsperson, but unfortunately only in the sense of traveling toward potential trouble. Still, as June says, "I know exercising with someone else is the smartest thing to do, but if it's a matter of either doing it alone or not doing it at all, I do it alone. But I do it the way I'd handle a porcupine . . . *very* carefully."

IDENTITY CRISIS

One of the basics for a diabetic, especially a physically active one, is some kind of identification showing that he or she *is* a diabetic. Because of a well-organized radio and TV public service campaign, people are becoming increasingly aware of Medic Alert bracelets and are starting to look for them in emergency situations. To our minds they are better than a wallet card. They can be seen more readily and—sad to state about the inhumanity of human nature these days—if a person is unconscious, that wallet well may disappear before help arrives.

Some diabetics prefer to wear their diabetic identification around their necks like dog tags. This isn't a bad idea, either, since if you are found unconscious your rescuer may open your collar, check your heartbeat, and so on, and a necklace diabetic identification is very likely to be noticed. In certain sports, though, like basketball or certain track and field events and swimming, a diabetic identification around the neck might be a distraction, if not an actual hazard. And it's not a good idea to wear the kind of identification you have to keep taking off. You might forget to put it on again and thereby blow the whole purpose of the diabetic identification—to have it on at all times, even when you sleep or shower.

Certain diabetics who don't want to be just half safe double up on their I.D.—for example, the bicyclist who not only wears a Medic Alert necklace but also has his bike marked that he is a diabetic. One long-distance runner we talked to teams a Medic Alert bracelet with an additional medical identification on the stopwatch he carries with him.

This is one area in which overkill *is* recommended. In a crisis a diabetic just can't have too much identity. For information about Medic Alert write:

> Medic Alert Foundation
> Turlock, California   95380

CASH AND CARRY

Pennies from heaven—and, more to the point, nickels and dimes and quarters—can't be counted on when a diabetic needs to buy emergency rations or preventive snacks or regular meals. Always carry both change for drink and candy machines and bills for bigger food purchases. (Is there no end to the things a diabetic has to carry around? Apparently not.)

If you let yourself get caught, with your pants empty of money, you may have to resort to the solution of a diabetic who has "gone into a café and ordered food, and eaten it even though I did not have any money, and when I got my blood sugar under control, I was able to talk my way out of it. . . . This is most embarrassing." (And here's another case in which diabetes identification would be very important—to help establish your excuse for putting a meal on the cuff.)

It isn't just food that you need money for, either. Coins can be the open sesame to pay-toilet doors when you need to test. June also sometimes uses the privacy of these booths for taking her before-meal injection.

Transportation to get you off your feet and home to your insulin or meal also costs money. Again, exact change is important. Once in Laguna Beach, California, June's blood sugar was beginning to wind down from her two-mile therapeutic walk, so she thought she'd take the bus back to where she was staying. She had to think again. She had only a $20 bill and the bus company, to thwart robberies, had a rule that you had to have exact change. This was a residential area with no change-making shops. She ended up doing the slowest mile walk on the record book in order not to bring on the impending reaction.

DOUBLE, DOUBLE TO AVOID TROUBLE

When you're backpacking and are going to be away from civilization for several days, you need to double up on both the diabetic vitals—insulin and food. If you take along an extra supply of insulin plus needles and testing material, then if one set of supplies is lost, *all* is not lost.

Naturally, you should get someone else to carry the extras. This is not a matter of lightening your load. Diabetic supplies don't weigh all that much—and, besides, you can carry something of your companion's. No, the reason you want someone else to carry the duplicate supplies is so that what engineers call the redundancy factor will then be in effect. Suppose a bear gets your pack and destroys it. If all the diabetic paraphernalia is in one place, it's all gone. This once happened to Dave Engerbretson in the woods. Fortunately, Dave's duplicates were in his wife's pack.

A pack can be lost or destroyed in many ways. It can get dropped in a river or knocked over a cliff (presumably when it's not attached to you) or stolen by marauding brigands—and who knows what other freaky things can happen to it?

ENOUGH IS NOT ENOUGH

The Boy Scout's motto, "Be prepared," is not enough for diabetics who participate in outdoor sports. Their motto has to be "Be overprepared." A Boy Scout whose preparation turned out to be inadequate might spend a cold and hungry night in the wilderness. A diabetic in the same circumstances could spend eternity there.

The time when you have to concern yourself the most with having plenty of blood-sugar raisers along is —obviously—when you're involved in a sport that gets you away from the Coke and candy machines of civilization. This includes sports such as skiing (both downhill and cross-country), hiking, backpacking, camping, canoeing, hunting and fishing, biking on country roads, mountain and rock climbing, and spelunking. (Cave explorers are probably the least likely to find a Coke machine at their elbow!)

When we asked outdoors-minded diabetics what they did if they were exercising heavily and found they didn't bring along enough food, we got such responses as:

"I have never been in this position, because I normally carry enough food for two persons!"

"Diabetics can never take the chance of being stranded without a source of sugar. Their life depends on it and there is no excuse for being careless on sports where you know there is a likelihood of being stranded —i.e., long lift lines for skiing, bike riding in the country."

Or, simply, "I don't see any solution when you don't bring enough food," and, "That is an error that can't be allowed to happen."

And yet sometimes it does happen. Dave Engerbretson's story of his spelunking adventure takes the cake, as well as any other high-carbohydrate product you can mention. He was exploring a cave in southern Indiana with some friends. From looking at a map they were reasonably certain that there was another entrance to the cave, and they were trying to find that second entrance.

They had been wandering around in the cave for some time when all of a sudden it dawned on Dave that he was almost out of food. Without food there was no way he was going to make it out of that cave. What had happened was that when they'd reached the point where they had to decide whether to turn back or to keep looking for the new entrance, they'd decided to go on. "That was when I blew it," said Dave. "That's when I should have realized that I only had enough food to get myself back out, and I shouldn't have gone on." But he did go on, and he ate all the food that was left.

Although he was in good shape at the moment, he knew that it wouldn't be long before the reaction would start. Since there didn't seem to be anything else to do, they turned around and started working their way back. But they weren't quite on the path they thought they were on. There were no marks on the walls or anything else to indicate that anyone had ever been in that part of the cave before. As they made their way along through the strange territory, Dave began to feel those old familiar sensations of insulin reaction. He had no idea what to do —except to say some prayers.

Finally they came to a small hole and, since it led off in the direction they wanted to go, they crawled through it on their bellies and found themselves in a huge room. Over in the corner they spotted something. Going over to

Preparations and Precautions

investigate, they found it was an old moldy rucksack. When they picked it up, it was so rotten it fell apart. Out tumbled a can of sardines and a can of peaches in heavy syrup. Dave's two buddies ate the sardines and Dave downed the whole can of peaches and, as he says, "lived happily ever after."

Dave considers that experience as close as he'll ever get to a miracle. But he blames himself for getting into such a position in the first place. "It was my own fault," he admits, "nobody else's. It was an error in judgment on my part, and diabetics can't afford to make errors in judgment."

Obviously, you can't always rely on a miracle. God, according to the cliché, helps those who help themselves, and the best way to help yourself is to be overprepared, with more food than is possibly required. Even on a one-day outing overpreparation is necessary. As one hiker explains it, "If I'm going into a remote area where the possibility exists of becoming lost or delayed, I take enough food to last at least twenty-four hours—in other words, enough to get me through the time period provided by the last insulin treatment."

A MOVABLE FEAST

We've been emphasizing the problem of running out of food in the wilderness, but you can have the same problem when you're only a short distance from home if there's no way to *get* home. This happened to a skier in Massachusetts who was driving home from the slopes. The road became so slippery that it was closed while they tried to get the sand trucks in. The normally ten-minute drive stretched into hours of sitting and waiting. It was the skier's dinnertime. Did she panic? Did she pass out? No, she did neither, because she always keeps crackers and peanut butter in her car, and on ski weekends she adds fruit to this storehouse, just in case what *did* happen happens. So she just ate and waited calmly for the trucks to arrive.

"Had I not anticipated problems such as this," she says, "I definitely would have been in a great deal of trouble, as there was no way to get food. This type of thinking becomes automatic and really is necessary for a diabetic to get used to."

EAT BEFORE YOU LEAP

You can't count on anything these days. All the Great Truths are crumbling before our eyes. For example, all our lives we've heard the Great Truth that toenails should be cut straight across, but now when June goes to her podiatrist for her regular diabetic foot maintenance, what does he do but shape—mind you, *shape*—the nail on her great toe, as the British call it. Is nothing sacred?

Nothing is, it seems, because another of life's Great Truths is going down the drainpipe as far as diabetics are concerned. We refer to the one about not exercising right after a meal. We both can remember stern parental admonitions to rest at least an hour or so after a meal so your stomach can have all the use of the blood for its big digestion project. Severe cramps and/or nausea were held out as the negative rewards of ignoring this advice. In the case of swimming, the predicted result of not waiting until at least an hour after eating was a little more

Preparations and Precautions 107

disastrous. The moment you hit the water, according to legend, you would double up with stomach cramps, sink out of sight, and drown yourself quite dead.

And so it happens that most of us have acquired a revulsion going on terror about exercising after a meal. Then along comes diabetes, a condition in which for insulin takers the very safest time to exercise is right after a meal. What are you to do? Most of the active diabetic sportspeople ignore the "don't-exercise-after-a-meal" edict. And well they should, because the truth of the matter is that the safest time for anyone to exercise is when the blood sugar is on the rise. Blood sugar reaches its height one to one and a half hours after a meal.

One basketball player's main problem in this respect has been bucking his teammates' reaction: "Ever since I became a diabetic and have had to eat snacks before practice, other guys have always bugged me and kidded me when they've seen me eating, and they've marveled at how I can eat so much and then practice without throwing up and getting sick. At first it used to bother me (the kidding) but it doesn't anymore. I just laugh and joke about it with them. And when they ask how I do it without getting sick, I just tell them I've got a cast-iron stomach."

Not that some diabetics don't have trouble with eating before practicing their sport, but it's usually an emotional rather than a physical problem—as in the case of our Maryland linebacker: "You are so uptight about the game and have a funny feeling inside and it's really hard to get anything down, especially when you know you are going out there to hit and be hit!"

Professor Leete says he runs "usually *immediately*

after a medium lunch of soup, meat sandwich, and canned fruit. I have never experienced discomfort or cramps from running immediately after a meal."

We've come up with a couple of opinions from other sources that both verify Professor Leete's experience and justify our linebacker's unsettled feeling. Wynn Updyke and Perry Johnson, in *Principles of Modern Physical Education, Health, and Recreation* (New York, Holt, Rinehart and Winston, Inc., 1970), write:

> It is not wise to eat just before or immediately following an activity that involves emotions or nervousness—for example, competitive athletics. This type of activity tends to interfere with the digestive process; however, *mild* exercise, not involving competition or emotions, is not harmful and may even act as an aid to digestion.

And UCLA exercise expert Lawrence Morehouse, in exploding the myth that swimming after eating is ruinous, says that "the traditionally feared cramps don't seem to be related to food at all—and have never caused drowning. I knew one American swimmer who ate a hamburger and four candy bars just before a 1968 Olympic race and then broke her own world's record.

"This is not to suggest that you eat a Thanksgiving dinner before swimming in a race. Any violent activity after a meal can cause nausea. But you can paddle around a warm pool to your heart's content."

MOUNTAIN HIGH, SUGAR LOW

We hate to keep strumming the same old banjo string over and over, but there is *no time* an insulin-taking diabetic can go out for exercise without emergency rations, even with preventive snacking beforehand. Here is a skier's story that makes a perfect object lesson.

"Baldy Mountain at Sun Valley even frightens me a little in the summer. When I first skied it I psyched myself very carefully. I skied the lower runs, becoming familiar with them. I then ate a whole candy bar and got on the lift feeling well fortified for whatever was ahead. About halfway down I had an insulin reaction. I lost my equilibrium and kept falling and coming out of my bindings.

"In sweeping the hill to close it, the ski patrol came upon me and was very nice and extremely patient with me. In spite of the fact that I was skiing with a friend who tried to explain to them what was happening, I overheard one say to the other, 'She is drunk.' My daughter (a diabetic) finally walked up to where I was, gave me a candy bar, and I skied down.

"I learned two things from this experience: (1) even though I had just eaten sugar before the run I should always have a reserve with me; and (2) although I was responsible for what happened, the ski patrol didn't seem to have the foggiest notion of what was going on. If either of us had had sugar, this could have been avoided."

This skier is not alone in her misadventure, at least not in the part about being accused of being drunk by the ski patrol. We had two other diabetics who were thought by the ski patrol to be under the influence. One reason for this is that there are probably a lot more drunks than diabetics on the slopes. It would seem, however, that part of the ski patrol's training should include the recognition of insulin shock. We wrote a letter of inquiry to the National Headquarters of the ski patrol in

Denver asking about their policy on this. They wrote back to say they were forwarding our letter to the proper person to answer. The proper person has not (as of this writing) done so. Undaunted, we talked to one of the P.E. men at the college where we work. He is Lynn Lomen, ski instructor and former patrol member. He said that, while there is no specific special training on recognizing insulin shock, each patrol member is required to take a first aid course—and insulin shock is covered in that.

The problem is, though, the one that we've mentioned previously. Lynn said that patrol members pick up drunks—and other mind-altering-drug users—so much more frequently than diabetics that, when they find someone staggering and slurring and falling down, their first reaction is *not* to go for carbohydrate.

When we asked about whether or not ski patrol members always check for Medic Alert bracelets or necklaces, he said, "They're supposed to, but when all clues point to drink or drugs sometimes they don't."

We asked if it would help if at the beginning of the day a diabetic went to the ski patrol hut and made his presence known. Lynn said it would help a *great deal.* Not only would the patrol members be alerted to the possibility of a diabetic's having a reaction on the slopes, but it would also probably inspire them to check their first aid manual and refresh their memories on the subject of diabetic emergencies. (Here's another situation in which a diabetic can help out his fellow "sweet pees," as one diabetic humorist calls them.)

Lynn went on to suggest that *any time* a diabetic practices a sport alone he should inform someone in authority of what to do in an emergency. For example, if you're out doing a round of golf on your own, tell the starter. If you're practicing your tennis serve by yourself, tell the playground director or tennis pro or whoever's in charge.

GIBSON GIRL

Another solution for diabetic skiers who want to be safe without taking any precautions themselves is to go ski Gibson Pass in British Columbia. There, we are informed, "the ski patrol has to be the most knowledgeable crew on diabetes there is."

Our informant, whose name is Laila Campbell, should know; she helped make them that way. She skis Monday through Friday. On a good day she gets in up to twenty-one runs. Since she's a brittle diabetic and problems could develop on the slopes, the ski patrol members at her area have all been instructed in how to administer the glucagon she carries at all times. She calls the ski patrol her "ever-loving conscience," because they keep an eye on her and even suggest rest breaks if she appears to be overdoing. Even so, she says, "Sometimes I have gone into a bad reaction and as a result had a fall into some rather weird positions and places."

Not only did the ski patrol extricate Laila Campbell from these weird positions and places, they were also kind enough to offer us some information on the problems they encounter with diabetics and some cautionary advice.

"One of the major symptoms experienced during shock is the respiratory problem. Breathing has to be checked at least every five minutes during transport to the patrol hut. Other factors further influence the respiratory problem. One of the biggest problems is deep powder snow. After falling in deep snow the diabetic usually has no energy and therefore remains buried until dug out. Even after transport to the patrol hut, it is very common for us to administer mouth-to-mouth A.R. for short periods.

"Another serious problem arises when a diabetic goes into shock while skiing. On one occasion Laila was found wedged into a 'bottomless' tree well. She wasn't found for three quarters of an hour, and it was extremely difficult to remove her because of possible back injuries. It is particularly difficult to diagnose injuries when the patient is unconscious, so one must be *extremely* cautious. Many of these problems could be prevented if diabetics restricted themselves to the *main* ski runs!"

SNACK PACK

When it comes to snacks for preventive maintenance and for catching insulin reactions in the early stages, most diabetic sportspeople carry along a few of their favorite things. These are usually chosen because they are not bulky and don't melt—not that taste is neglected, though. Most diabetics select something they enjoy. As one says, "It is really the only time to have a sweet of some kind, and you never really lose your sweet tooth." Others agree. "When my blood sugar is low from exercise I can have a little treat like cake or candy that I normally could not have if my blood sugar was normal."

Preparations and Precautions

Bobby Clarke, who needs a good solid carbohydrate hype for his high-energy sport as a Philadelphia Flyer, is a Coke man. He downs one before each game and another during each period.

One cross-country skier and hiker packs "peanut butter and marmalade sandwiches on rich bread (banana or apple sauce) in winter for more calories for ski touring. Besides being quick to make, peanut butter sandwiches don't spoil in the heat or freeze in the cold." Since ski touring and hiking demand lots of restorative food, she also carries "candy, cookies, and dried fruit. In summer gumdrop-type candy seems to slide down most easily (and doesn't melt in the pack). In winter we carry 'gorp,' a mixture of nuts, chocolate bits, raisins, currants, and other dried fruit cut up—the recipe varies among individuals—a case of *chacun à son gorp!*"

A gymnast munches Chuckles, "which can be chewed up quickly and are about twenty calories a chuck, so I can measure the amount I eat. Also, they don't melt, so when you dig into the bottom of your bag you don't come up with any liquid matter."

Another diabetic is a devotee of brownies. "For an extremely strenuous sport, such as skiing, I normally eat a brownie before starting. . . . I have found that a brownie is the best food available to take prior to skiing because of its sugar, carbohydrate, and milk content. This has been confirmed by several doctors that I discussed it with. At first they are surprised that I eat brownies, but then realize it is the best source for the additional requirement needed by the body for both short term (sugar needed immediately) and long term (additional sugar needed by the body after skiing for a long period)."

You can see the combination of short term (concentrated sugar) and long term (slower-acting carbohydrates and proteins) in this random list of favorite snacking things mentioned by diabetic sports and exercise enthusiasts.

apples
bananas
beef jerky
Breakfast Squares
cheese and crackers
chewing gum
chocolate-covered wafers
Chunkies
cookies
cupcakes
dried fruit
Good and Plenty
graham crackers
junior baby food (especially pureed fruit)
M&M's
maple sugar candy
milk
nuts
peanut butter crackers
potato chips
raisin-peanut-chocolate snack
Spacefood Sticks
sweet rolls
Tic-Tacs
Tootsie Rolls
various sandwiches

The list goes on, but maybe this much will give you some new snacking ideas or at least open your mind to the idea that diabetic treatment can be a treat. (For the sugar content of various blood-sugar-raising snacks, see Appendix F.)

The only difficulty that may present itself when you're always prepared with a good supply of tasty snacks is that they may be just a little too tempting. "At one time I carried a prescription vial filled with M&M's," explains a sixteen-year-old sportswoman, "but I found that I was snacking on them when it wasn't necessary." So here's another line for the diabetic to walk: carrying a snack

Preparations and Precautions 115

that's good enough to make you want to eat it when you need it, yet not so good that you can't resist it when you don't need it.

FUELISH NOTIONS

A question put to us by several insulin takers concerned whether it is preferable before all-day activities to depend on high-carbohydrate snacks or high-protein meals. Long runs, bike rides, hikes, and skiing especially bring up this question of the best food fuel. We went to Dr. Olson for the answer to this one and this is what he said:

"Proteins are not a very good source of immediate energy under any circumstances; really, the two best sources of energy are carbohydrates first and then fats. Carbohydrates are used for short spurts of energy until the supply is exhausted, and then fats are brought into use to furnish calories for physical expenditure. The advantage of proteins, of course, is the fact that 58 percent of protein can be made into sugar by gluconeogenesis and thus furnish a longer supply of available carbohydrate.

"I advise my people who are going on day-long bike tours or backpacking, etc., simply to have six meals a day: breakfast; a good midmorning snack consisting of both protein and carbohydrates, like a peanut butter sandwich and a glass of milk; usual lunch; good afternoon snack; usual supper; and bedtime snack. This is the same advice I give to the diabetic farmer who is out in the fields all day long. On such a program they may run a little glucosuria, but this is not going to get them into any trouble, as would severe hypoglycemia."

WITH FRIENDS LIKE THIS . . .

We're always advocating that a diabetic never do his or her sports thing alone. But we admit that sometimes your companions can be hazardous to your health. This is when they munch away your Life Savers, both literally and figuratively. Some diabetics report that others are always eating up their snacks. One even complains that, when he's engaged in sports, "The managers always eat my Life Savers or sugar cubes."

What to do? Well, you can give them lengthy lectures on the problems of diabetes and how you need these emergency rations to counteract the effects of your insulin. Or you can give them a karate chop each time their paws venture toward your snack supply. Or you can use a more amiable although more expensive method: "I usually carry far more food than I need, but it certainly makes me popular with friends when they are starved and I have all sorts of snacks handy."

The problem is a little tougher when it's a matter of lunch out on the trail or up on a rock or down in a cave, as one hiker explains: "I have sat on the mountaintop eating my lunch while a companion watched without food because he was too lazy to carry a lunch, trying to explain, of course, that my full lunch was a matter of necessity with me."

This predicament is especially hard if, like a good, prudent diabetic, you have brought along double food supplies to cover an emergency. It's going to be doubly tough to explain to a starving friend why you can't spare him or her a carrot stick, let alone a ham sandwich, when you obviously have two whole lunches in your pack.

Preparations and Precautions 117

The trick here is to explain not *then* but before the outing. Tell your friend—and make sure the message is getting through—that you *have* to eat all the food you bring for lunch and you *have* to save food for an emergency. Explain what will happen if you don't eat all you're supposed to. Paint a vivid word picture of the struggle to carry or drag your limp (but leaden) body out of the wilderness. Convince your friend that it is imperative to bring a complete and separate lunch or bear the consequences of a growling stomach and low blood sugar. (Yes, nondiabetics can have low blood sugar, too, but it usually just makes them tired and mean, e.g.: "You !@#$%¢&. You could at least let me have a !@#$%¢& apple out of that !@#$%¢& ten-course lunch of yours!")

Or, if you happen to be a (check one) ☐ Samaritan ☐ sucker, you could just capitulate and follow the aforementioned surefire method and make an extra lunch for your friend. But at least see that the !@#$%¢& carries it—not you.

COOL IT

"I would like to go on extended backpacking and canoeing trips, but I haven't been able to figure a way of keeping my insulin chilled for a prolonged period. Any suggestions?" This is a common question among outdoor-minded insulin-taking diabetics.

Our suggestion is to cool it—meaning to cool your worries, *not* your insulin. If it's an old wives' tale that you can't exercise after eating, it's an old pharmacists' tale that you have to keep your insulin refrigerated. (We suspect that it's the tale of a foxy old pharmacist who wants to sell you one of those expensive special little insulin-keeping thermos bottles.)

Now hear this—and please believe it. Unless you're doing your hiking and camping at high noon in midsummer in Death Valley, you don't have to worry about keeping your insulin cool. A doctor once told us that one of the drug companies, by way of experiment, kept a bottle of insulin sitting out on a shelf at room temperature for several years and when they tested it it was still OK. A nurse once explained that insulin is like your hand. You wouldn't boil it and you wouldn't freeze it, but otherwise it can take any temperature you can without damage.

Sometimes, in an effort to keep insulin cool, you can do it more harm than good. One diabetic we talked to at a diabetes association meeting told us that once, when he was flying to Hawaii, he put his insulin into a wide-mouthed thermos and packed ice around it. By the time he was on the ground again with a lei around his neck the insulin was frozen and ruined and had to be thrown away.

Freezing is the really bad thing for insulin. High temperatures merely cause it to diminish slightly in effectiveness. If avoiding freezing is the problem, how about ski tourers and snow campers? What are they to do to keep their insulin from freezing? Easy. When June is ski touring, she keeps her insulin in an inside pocket where it's warmed by the body's central heating system. On freezing nights just keep it with you inside the sleeping bag. You can even take your shot there in cozy comfort and privacy the way Dave Engerbretson does—well, not *quite* the way he does, since, as he reports about insulin taking, "I've done it inside a sleeping bag when I couldn't see what I was doing and stuck the darn thing in my finger."

FOOT NOTE

We hate to add to the annals of diabetes yet another harangue about "the diabetic foot," but we do feel there should be a few well-chosen words on the subject, especially for sportspeople. Since nobody chooses words better than Thom Underwood, let's hear his advice:

"No bare feet. I'm a fanatic about my feet. Mostly because in all my hobbies, all the best parts of my life, I use them. Blisters and such cause nothing but problems and pain and destroy the pleasure. Clean socks, foot powder, and moleskin prevent a problem before it starts."

We might add that the shoes you wear are also problem preventers, if you get the right kind. For sports—including walking—shoes are particularly important. They should be fitted carefully, and you should be willing to spend a few dollars on them. Limp tennies that have been through the washer a dozen times provide neither support nor protection. It's a far better plan to spend a little more, or—let's be realistic—quite a lot more on quality sports shoes such as those made by Adidas, Tretorn, or Tiger. They will last longer and help your feet last longer as well.

Another worthwhile investment is an occasional trip to the podiatrist or, if you have any continuing foot problems, regular trips to the podiatrist. Podiatrists are highly trained people who know what they are doing. They must complete four years of podiatry college on top of at least two years of undergraduate work, although most of them have their four-year B.A. or B.S. degrees.

Unfortunately, people are still confusing them with the chiropodists of yore who used to hang out a shingle after about fifteen minutes of instruction—or none at all. As one podiatrist told us, podiatry is now in the same position as dentistry was about seventy-five years ago: it is struggling for recognition as a skilled profession. If you want to be sure of getting a qualified podiatrist, write to the American Podiatry Association, 20 Chevy Chase Circle, N.W., Washington, D.C. 20015, for a list of those in your area.

Now, after these words of podiatric encouragement, a few words of caution. Since podiatrists *are* highly trained professionals, what they seem to most enjoy doing is highly trained professional-type work, i.e., surgery. It has happened to both of us that when we've gone to a podiatrist for some minor but irritating and possibly painful problem like soft corns or callus buildup, the podiatrist has told us that surgery is the only permanent cure. He has said that anything else is just "first aid" and won't last more than a few weeks or months. We believe this; yet for both of us, but especially for June of the diabetic feet, the idea of something as major as minor surgery to get rid of calluses doesn't make sense and *does* make our hair stand on end and our toes curl. Consequently, June makes it clear that first aid is all she's after. Once the podiatrist accepts this aberration, she has a fine, long range, regular relationship with him. She also has feet that cause her no trouble at all.

While we're on the subject of feet and athletes, it is only natural that our thoughts should turn toward ath-

Preparations and Precautions 121

lete's foot. Everybody knows that, despite the name, this fungus infection is not restricted to Olympic team members and Heisman Trophy winners. Everybody may not know, however, that—again despite its name—athlete's foot is not restricted to the feet. It involves the whole body and can lead to serious complications, including that old nemesis of all diabetics, gangrene.

Athlete's foot should not be treated lightly. It *should* be treated promptly. We heard Southern California diabetes association official Dr. Russell Poucher recommend the use of Tinactin if you catch athlete's foot in its early stages. You can get this without prescription from your friendly neighborhood druggist. If you let it go without treatment about six months or so, you get nail involvement. At this stage, Dr. Poucher recommends Fulvicin. This is a prescription drug, though, so in order to get it you have to consult your doctor, who may have his own ideas on the treatment. Suffice it to say that it will be a lot less hard on your system—and your pocketbook—if you treat athlete's foot while it's still in its beginning stages.

4

A Mature Attitude

One thing you notice about many maturity-onset diabetics is that you *don't* notice them. You don't notice them being really careful about their diets or really regular in their exercise routines. This is, we suspect, because they don't really take their diabetes seriously. When you're a juvenile-onset diabetic sticking the needle in yourself every day, you get the point that you are a diabetic, and you know you'd jolly well better act the part.

Maturity onsets, however, often consider themselves "mild" or "borderline" and figure they can have a more casual approach to diabetes care. This wrong figure can get them into more trouble than a wrong figure on an income tax form. As the pioneer of diabetes care, Dr. Elliott Joslin, put it, "the mild case neglected almost always becomes severe."

Mind you, we're not saying that *all* maturity-onset diabetics act as if they don't have it. Some are as conscientious as any juvenile-onset who ever filled a syringe. We came in contact with two particularly shining examples, and we hope that presenting their life-styles will encourage other maturity-onsetters to go and do likewise.

PORTRAIT OF A PILL TAKER

June Albert takes two tablets of Orinase a day and two of D.B.I. (these pills lower blood sugar). June has the distinction of being that incongruity of the diabetes world, a young pill taker. She's only twenty-four. In our opinion, though, it's quite possible that without her attention to exercise and diet she wouldn't be distinctive at all. She'd be just another classic young insulin-dependent diabetic.

June lives in Wolcott, Connecticut, and works there as a full-time junior accountant in a bank—a job with a lot of responsibility—and attends a university part-time in pursuit of her accounting degree. Eventually she expects to become a C.P.A.

"I have only known about my diabetes for one year," June told us. "I was born a natural athlete, I guess, and have always been proud of my sports ability and my health in general. It was an emotional blow to realize I had diabetes, an incurable disease." Because June was determined to show herself she could still do everything she wanted to in spite of her diabetes, she read every book she could find on the subject and attended a one-week five-hour class in diabetes education.

Since her doctor knew she was very active and engaged in sports, he gave her a 2,000-calorie-a-day diet, which is on the high side (she's 5 feet 4 inches and weighs 115 pounds). But she says she does eat about that much every day.

Her regulation of her diabetes is exceptionally good. "In the year I've been on pills I've never spilled, except for one time, that I know of. This was because I forgot to take my medicine for a whole day and my diet wasn't exactly correct that day, either. I check my urine about twice a week. I know it should be more often."

June says she probably messes up with her diet more than with getting her exercise or taking her medication. This she attributes to being so busy that she sometimes can't eat enough of what she should or exactly everything that's on her diet. "Sometimes I don't have a vegetable when I should, but I don't substitute anything wrong like bread for the vegetable. I hardly ever eat something that's forbidden like candy or anything with sugar in it. If I do, it's always when I've had to go without eating for much longer than I should, which hardly ever happens."

Because she doesn't need insulin June doesn't feel regulated in her activities, only in her diet. One thing that has changed is that now she plays sports around her eating schedule of three regular meals and three snacks. Before her diabetes she used to eat when convenient. Now, however, she goes right home after work and has her meal, while maybe the easier thing would be to go to her health spa or play tennis before going home to eat. According to June, "That's the only problem—making time to eat."

She also finds she has to alter her diet plan some on days when she plays tennis or rides her bike. She saves part of her lunch or supper and eats it just before she plays tennis or rides, but she's emphatic on one point: "I don't eat extra food."

June doesn't think of her sports participation as having much to do with her diabetes. No, she looks to sports as a way to socialize, keep in shape, compete, learn about herself, and relax, all at the same time. Because of the er-

A Mature Attitude

ratic climate she lives in, she changes her sports activities to match the weather. She enjoys that, because she loves variety.

"Tennis I play once or twice a week in summer and occasionally in the winter," June says. "Bike riding is occasionally and only in the spring, summer, and fall, but usually for long distances like ten to twenty miles. Swimming—I probably swim one mile a week all year round, because I belong to a health spa and I go there once or twice a week and sometimes three times a week."

Those are her regular sports. In the winter she ice skates about once a month and is learning to ski, too. She tries to go twice a month for weekend trips.

June's most regular exercise—it's not at all seasonal—is going to her health spa. Her program of exercise there changes every two months, because this is their policy. She works on the needed areas of tightening or fitness, measures her progress, and changes the exercises accordingly. She does routine exercises for one half hour, jogs fifteen minutes, jogs outside for one mile in good weather or swims one mile in the pool. Sometimes she winds up with a few swimnastics in the pool.

June's other way of getting regularity into exercise is to walk up and down stairs at work rather than using the elevator. Usually she also walks for half an hour at lunchtime to walk off her meal.

June engaged in most all her sports before she knew she was diabetic, but they took on a different, more important meaning in her life afterward. "I guess before sports were something to do with my leisure time and to stay in shape. Now I'm concerned with staying in shape and feeling good *primarily*. My goals have changed. I'm more determined to live a full and healthy life as long as I can. I'm *much* more competitive in sports now. I want to prove to myself that *I can do it,* if it's beating someone better than me at tennis or running longer and faster than my seventeen-year-old sister (who's a good athlete).

"Because I try harder now and I'm curious about my limits, I have really accomplished much more than I ever would have thought I could. This makes me thankful, because I've gained so much confidence through sports that helps me in my career. That's the most important thing about sports to me—the change in my outlook, in my attitude toward life."

DO AND DIET

We've already mentioned Shelly Lowenkopf, the forty-four-year-old diet-and-exercise-controlled diabetic who is a sedentary editor. Or rather, his work is sedentary. He is ambulatory in the extreme, if you call getting up at 4:30 A.M. to ambulate extreme—and we do! Diabetes has made Shelly into a walker and a runner.

In the beginning Shelly's outing was just fast-paced walking in the unpaved netherworld of Mulholland Drive high above Los Angeles. He pushed for four or five miles a day and, as muscles appeared, upped things to six, seven, and finally ten.

"By this point," says Shelly, "I felt perfectly self-righteous because none of my clothing would fit and the M.D. had upped me to 2,200 calories per day. Food tasted better, I seemed to require less of it at a sitting, work output was much more prolonged. Rewards along the way: went from a 36-inch waist and 195 pounds to a more realistic 33 waist and 165 pounds."

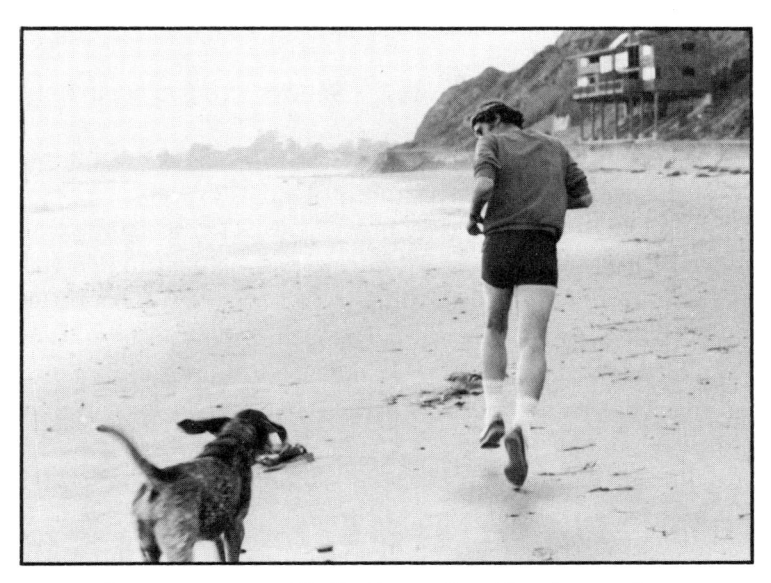

Every day you can see Shelly Lowenkopf by the seashore running his dogs—and normal blood sugar.

Shelly was so pleased with his new self that he gradually changed his walking beat into a run. First he'd run one mile, then two, then three, until all ten of his miles were running miles. His ambition now is to get into the marathon class, and he's looking forward to his first race.

"Exercise," he says, "is important to me now because I realize how good I feel when I do it regularly. I resent the things during the course of a day which cut into the exercise, and I tend to get bitter and grouchy when I have to miss a day. Used to be the shower was the place where I did all my high-powered thinking, such as preparing lectures for my classes or reviewing the day's writing stint or the day's work problems. But now there is something nearly metaphysical about running for me, whether it is on a track, the grassy parkway at Santa Barbara's East Beach, or the beach itself. I won't run on sidewalks or streets anymore, because I once in the throes of investigating some flight of fancy ran into a parked car."

Shelly told us that a noted Los Angeles physician, Ronald A. Lawrence—himself a runner—has estimated that an athlete in his or her prime, in top competing condition for the Olympics, will lose all muscle tone and conditioning in thirty days if there is not a constant training program. The doctor has also estimated that prolonged slow exercise is the answer to maintaining the best possible cardiovascular and muscle conditioning. So, as Shelly says, "The messages start coming through: If you don't use it, you lose it. If you lose it, you're prey to the same life-shortening diseases and dysfunctional problems as non-diabetics, which is bad enough without your being more vulnerable than they. If you become a skinny, loose-muscled, fun-loving diabetic, you're going to be around and happy for a long time, baby, and that's winning, too."

Shelly's success story contains one cautionary note for non-insulin-taking diabetics who are overweight and starting out on an exercise program. His morning exercise routine became a trauma while he was losing weight and remetabolizing. His frequent dizzy spells in the midst of exercise made him less than eager to get up and out at so ungodly an hour as 4:30 A.M., but as soon as he got the idea of taking a snack along—usually some peanuts—the dizzy spells stopped and he began to look forward to the outing.

Since a diet-controlled diabetic who engages in an exercise program the likes of Shelly's can be susceptible to low-blood-sugar feelings, Shelly takes precautions just as an insulin taker would:

"I try to squirrel away (pun intended) caches of

raw peanuts or cashews. In a dire emergency a small can of unsweetened grapefruit juice. There is hardly a refrigerator to which I have any access that does not have bits of Tillamook or Brie or Camembert. My absolute favorite thing to have at hand in crisis is Laura Scudder's crunchy peanut butter, 'cause Laura don't mess wif no hydrogenated oils er none of that other specious gunk."

Shelly admits to becoming just as cranky as an insulin taker when he underestimates the amount of food he'll need on a run. The main difference between him and an insulin-taking diabetic is that he usually exercises before a meal rather than after.

EXERCISE, FOR CRIPE'S SAKE

That's all very well, you may say, for a twenty-four-year-old or a forty-four-year-old. But what if you're a fifty-four-year-old or a sixty-four-year-old or even a seventy-four-year-old? And what if you've never been much for sports and exercise and you're all out of shape and maybe you have a heart condition and possibly a touch of arthritis? What then?

Well, then it's time—high time—and it's definitely not too late to get yourself physically fit. You need to do this both for the sake of your diabetes and for the rest of your body's sake, too. To define that delightful condition known as physical fitness and to explain how to get it, we went to our physical education expert, Dave Engerbretson. Dave defined it as "having the ability to get through your normal daily living without undue fatigue and with enough reserve energy left to meet any unforeseen emergency." This means that each person has individual fitness requirements, which depend on an individual life-style. There is no one magic formula for everyone.

Incidentally, what you consider an emergency may be quite different from what an emergency is to your body. For instance, the body reacts to tennis on a weekend as an emergency. In other words, even having fun is an emergency to your body. That's why your life-style has a bearing on what the correct level of physical fitness is for you.

What are the unique components of physical fitness? These, Dave explained, were carefully isolated in a recent study at the University of Illinois, and they turned out to be strength, flexibility, agility, balance, power (how fast you perform), and endurance. If you are fit in all six of these factors, then you can consider yourself to have total physical fitness.

The method Dave outlined was a way to become fit and at the same time to become a more active, well-controlled diabetic. Basically, the program is built around cardiovascular fitness—your heart, blood vessels, respiration, and circulation. But, again, if it's strength, flexibility, agility, or any of the other six individual components of fitness that you need, you can develop those, too. Dave calls the method "continuous, rhythmical, interval, progressive, endurance training," because each of those words tells you something about the program. He put the words in that order because they spell CRIPE, which is easier to remember. Here is what each of these words refers to in the context of an exercise program.

CONTINUOUS—This means that the exercise must be done continuously without stopping. If you're going to exercise for half an hour, you don't stop once during that entire half hour.

RHYTHMICAL—A rhythmical exercise is one in which the muscles are contracting and relaxing on a rhythmical basis. Walking, jogging, running, hiking, cross-country skiing, swimming, bicycle riding, rowing a boat—all these activities are rhythmical. You are moving yourself from one place to another under your own power in a steady manner. You can see that games like golf and tennis do not qualify—there is too much stop and go, which breaks up the rhythm.

INTERVAL—This word describes how you exercise continuously for your half hour or forty-five minutes or whatever. You work fast and then you alternate with an interval at a slower pace. Swim fast for two pool lengths, then slow for one; fast for two, slow for one, etc. By alternating speeds you can catch your breath enough not to have to stop completely.

PROGRESSIVE—This means that your exercise becomes progressively a little more difficult. When your body adjusts to one level of work load, then you increase the amount you do. The trick is to progress in a lot of little steps.

ENDURANCE—This word simply says that you're doing an endurance-type program, one that lasts more than five or ten minutes. Endurance activities improve your cardiovascular fitness, and that's the most important kind of fitness for a diabetic.

Now you're equipped with the theory behind the program you're going to be designing for yourself. It's the continuous, rhythmical, interval, progressive, endurance training. So how do you go about setting up your CRIPE program?

First, you have a physical examination and get checked out with your physician. Then you pick your activity. Choose something you personally enjoy doing— or at least don't despise doing. Let's say you've decided on jogging. You put on your comfortable jogging suit and your special running shoes and you go out and run until you feel a little winded. Then you slow down and walk until you've recovered. Then you jog again until your breath gives out. Jog, walk, jog, walk. You'll discover your interval this way. You may begin by jogging a block and walking a block. Somebody else may be able to start by jogging two blocks and walking only half a block. You serve as your own judge.

"Maybe you're eighty-five years old and you don't jog too well," said Dave. "Then your interval at first might be walk slowly a block and shuffle half a block."

He recommends to diabetics who want to be active that they do their CRIPE program three times a week and that the other days they play games—tennis, golf, or something similar—just for a change and also because diabetics should be quite regular. They should avoid doing a lot today and nothing tomorrow. Research has shown that the CRIPE program should be done at least an hour a day three days a week. In spite of what some of the best-selling books say, less than that isn't enough.

Even after you get into shape, according to Dave, you should always be tired when you stop your stint, but you should recover quickly. Here again you have to be your own judge and cut back if you need to.

You keep progressing until you get to the point where you want to stay. Incidentally, it takes less work to stay at a level of fitness than it does to get there in the first place. When you finally have all the energy you need for

A Mature Attitude

your daily life plus any unexpected emergencies, then you've hit your level. But if you quit it's right downhill again.

"If you keep at it," Dave promised, "your life's going to be a lot more enjoyable. We all know sixty-five-year-olds who are really old and other sixty-five-year-olds who have the vigor of forty-five-year-olds. The active sixty-five-year-olds are always out playing golf or going fishing and they can't find enough hours in the day to fit in all they want to do. These people are generally very happy people in spite of their age."

Dave went on to explain that you can develop the other six individual components of fitness by working some calisthenics into your program. We have found that fifteen minutes a day of calisthenics does great things for your shape. And in spite of the recent proliferation of newer-fangled programs, we stick to that old reliable that started the exercise craze in this country, the *Royal Canadian Air Force Exercise Plans for Physical Fitness*. We especially like its gradual method of progression.

DIFFERENT CRIPES FOR DIFFERENT TYPES

Although we used jogging as our CRIPE example and although some of the most passionately dedicated, not to say fanatic, diabetic sportspeople are runners, jogging and running are definitely not the only ways to go on an exercise program. In fact, we must admit that jogging and running bore the very sweatsuits off us. Try as we may, we have never managed to reach that mystic transcendental moment that runners rave about. It's always been a dull interminable thud, thud, thud, as far as we're concerned.

And we've always been sorely aware of the physical

problems of jogging as well as its documented physical benefits. Dick Bernstein's doctor wife told us of an article in the *Journal of the American Medical Association* that reported that 80 percent of long-term joggers develop jogger's knee. But according to Dick, you don't need to read the article to know that. Just look at a group of joggers and see how many are wearing knee bands.

Dr. Olson also has some reservations about the benefits of jogging. One of his doctor friends, an ardent and dedicated jogger, dropped dead one day in the midst of a jog. And that's just one of many such happenings Dr. Olson can report.

Now that we've absolved you of guilt feelings if jogging has never won your heart as a cardiovascular-improving activity, what are the alternatives? Swimming, of course, is one of the best, but it does require a rather large, nonportable piece of equipment. What we prefer are activities that can be done in the privacy of your own home or out your front door without a huge outlay of money. The three activities that to our minds meet these requirements are jumping rope, bicycling, and walking.

Getting the Jump on Health. A particularly fine all-round exercise for diabetics is jumping rope. It's a perfect CRIPE. You can get as much exercise in ten minutes of rope jumping as in thirty minutes of jogging. You can exercise both arms and legs. You can do it in any season, indoors and outdoors, and if you do it on a soft surface, you run less risk of damaging your knees and assorted cartilages than you do jogging on a hard surface.

Best of all, you don't even need a rope to jump rope. June discovered that she kept whacking herself in the shins when she jumped rope. This not only was an unpleasant sensation but it broke up the rhythm of the exercise. So she eliminated the problem—the rope. Now she jumps rapidly, rhythmically, and happily, going through each motion, including the arm swings, just as though the rope were there. (Her next idea is to learn to play golf without the ball, since that poisonous pellet is the one thing that louses up an otherwise perfect game.)

If you do decide to use the rope, you can go for one of those nifty professional models with ball bearings in the handles, or you can make it with No. 10 sash cord, which you can buy in almost any hardware store. Whatever kind of rope you use, though, make sure it's the right length. You should be able to stand with both feet on the rope and have it reach your armpits.

If you find it too strenuous to jump with both feet, use the one-foot-at-a-time-step-over method. If you find jumping rope not challenging enough, you can try doing it backwards. This not only reduces the boredom but improves rhythm and coordination.

Wheeling and Dealing. Biking has good associations with diabetes. Many areas of the United States have diabetes fund-raising bike rides, usually held with the cooperation of McDonald's restaurants. In these the riders have sponsors who agree to pay them so much for every mile they ride, and the proceeds go to the American Diabetes Association.

Bicycling also has good physical associations with diabetes. There's no activity better for keeping those tenuous lower extremities in good working order. Every time you push the pedal the muscles of your legs squeeze the blood vessels, helping return the blood to the heart. When you pump a bike you are literally pumping blood and improving circulation. It is for this reason that we recommend a ten-speed bike with some fairly low "Alpine" gears (in the upper thirties) or even granny gears (in the lower thirties). In case you're not familiar with bike gears, the lower the gear number, the more you pedal but the less effort it takes to push the pedal. Since you get more cardiovascular benefit from repeated pedaling than you do from muscling your way along in a high gear, we recommend riding in a gear five to ten points lower than the average cyclist would be riding in.

To make still another odious comparison with jogging, one active—*very* active—sixty-five-year-old gave up his favorite sport, jogging, in favor of his second favorite sport, biking, when he was sixty-four, because "you can train harder with the bicycle without getting the soreness and pain you get from jogging."

One of the best features of biking is that it's a CRIPE that can become a way of life. If you really get addicted, you can use your bike for your major transportation and kick the debilitating (both financially and physically) automobile habit. But even if you can't use a bike to eliminate the car, you can use it to add new dimensions to your life as you explore new scenes at a speed at which you can really see and experience them and acquire that wonderful sensation of freedom that getting around under your own power can bring.

You can get all the physical benefits of biking from a stationary bicycle exercise machine—but, alas, none of the esthetic and emotional ones.

Sole Food. And now we come to walking, another one of those best things in life that are free. Most people don't

A Mature Attitude

particularly consider walking a sport, but it is, or it can be if you do it enough and do it at a good clip. What's more, it's the one sport that virtually anyone can do without risk. In fact, as one doctor put it, "It's impossible to walk too much." And the Joslin Clinic unequivocally states in its manual, "Walking is the best exercise for your feet."

So don't scorn walking. It's a major part of June's exercise program. She tries to get in four miles a day. And if you'd like a more professional endorsement of walking, take Bill Talbert. On days when he doesn't play tennis, he makes it a point to walk forty to fifty blocks.

Now when we say walking, we don't mean just moseying and meandering, although that's certainly better than doing nothing. No, when we say walking, we mean briskly striding along with the ultimate goal of clicking

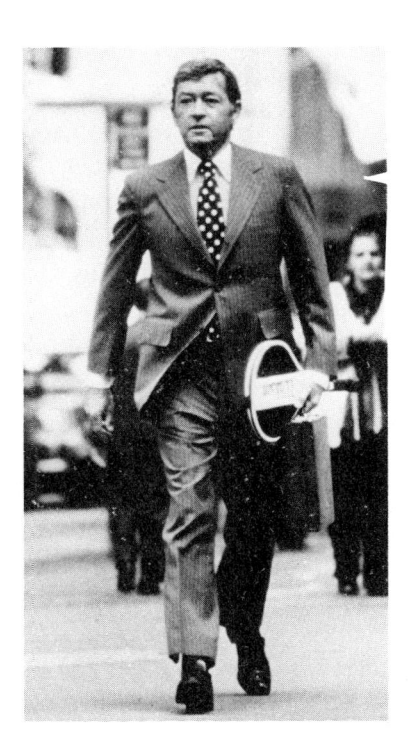

Bill Talbert, walking with a briefcase, a tennis racquet—and a purpose.
(Photo: Bill Ray)

off a fifteen-minute mile, a speed which will get you on the verge of a dogtrot.

If you get into serious walking, we recommend using a pedometer so you can know how far and fast you've gone and work toward a little farther and a little faster each day.

GRAY POWER

For the older diabetic—and we mean those who are between sixty-five and eighty-five—an exercise program to improve circulation to the lower extremities is a kind of insurance policy against the dire things that can happen to diabetic toes, feet, and legs in advanced years. And the first exercises we're going to recommend are so easy that anyone can do them. You perform them in your own bedroom in your pajamas. And, should you have a heart problem, there's no need for concern. (You see, there are absolutely *no* excuses for not doing these.)

Buerger-Allen Exercises. We were introduced to these little wonder exercises by physical therapist Roger C. Larson. He's done a lot of work with older diabetics, and, although he has dealt with some very active diabetics in their seventies who walked five to six miles a day, he has had others who claimed they could hardly walk at all because every time they walked they'd get decubitus ulcers on their heels. (Decubitus ulcers are bedsores, but they're not caused only by being in bed. They also appear wherever blood circulation is diminished.) Roger promises that by restoring the circulation in the lower extremities these exercises will get decubitus ulcers off your feet and you *on* your feet in only three to four weeks.

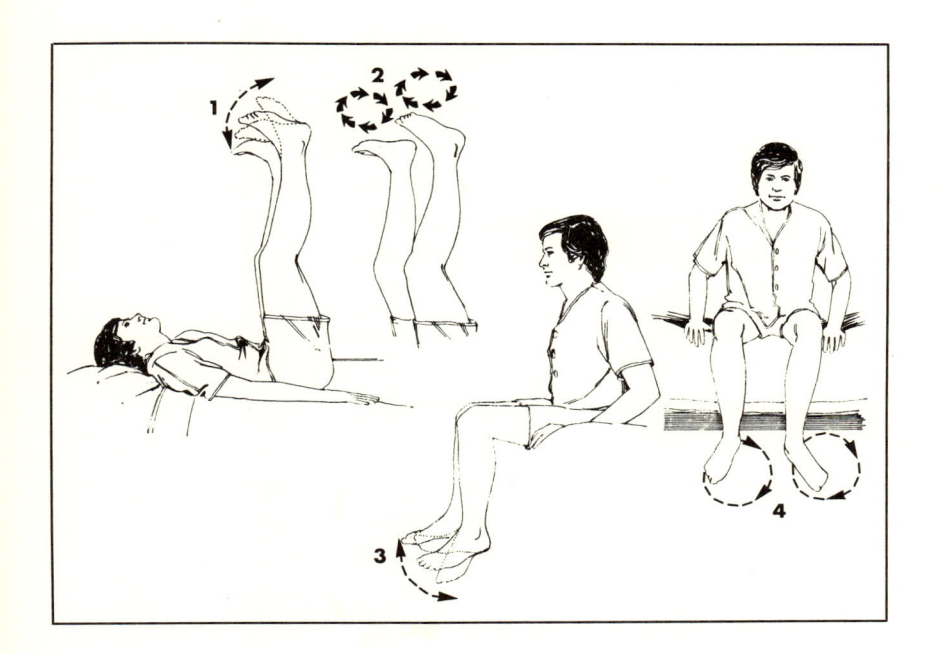

This routine is to be followed every morning, even when you are traveling or are a guest in someone's home. Perform them *before* you get out of bed. (Don't even go to the bathroom first, because getting up and walking around changes your metabolism.)

Exercise No. 1

Lying flat on your back, lift your legs until they are straight above your hips. From this position, with the soles of your feet facing the ceiling, move your feet up and down, bending them at the ankle, so that your toes are first pointing to the ceiling and then to the bed. Repeat ten to twelve times.

Exercise No. 2

While in the same position, make clockwise circles with your feet ten to twelve times. Then make counterclockwise circles ten to twelve times.

Exercise No. 3

Sit up and hang your legs over the edge of the bed, but don't touch the floor with your feet. Flex your ankles and point your toes first up, then down, as you did in Exercise 1. Do this ten to twelve times.

Exercise No. 4

Now, while in the same position, do the clockwise and counterclockwise circles you did in Exercise 2. Repeat ten to twelve times as before.

What the Buerger-Allen exercises do is get all the garbage out of your system from lying down all night. They also work wonders for leg aches, and they help to cure decubitus ulcers of the feet. If your ankles swell in the late afternoon, repeat the exercise series and you'll get some relief from that, too. Roger Larson guarantees that these simple exercises will also make you just plain feel better.

Dick's Trick: Bernsteins. The next step up from Buerger-Allen exercises are what we have come to call "Bernsteins," because we first learned about them from Dick Bernstein. Out of the entire exercise routine he performs daily, this is the one exercise he recommends for almost all diabetics, provided they do not have a history of retinal hemorrhages or coronary problems or thrombophlebitis (inflammation of a vein resulting in clot formation). It's an important exercise for diabetics because it improves the blood circulation in the feet and legs and also because it helps counteract the deterioration of the small blood vessels in the lower extremities. Dick cautions, however, that if a diabetic is over forty he should consult a doctor before beginning this program, because the heart rate and blood pressure go way up during the exercise.

A Mature Attitude 141

Dick considers the exercise especially valuable for pregnant diabetics and for elderly diabetics, because it helps prevent the buildup of fluids in the lower extremities. A fluid buildup is quite common in elderly diabetics and in even normal pregnancies, to say nothing of diabetic ones.

Dick says this exercise, if done intensively and repeatedly, can also put considerable strain on the heart and thereby increase the heart rate and build up stamina. On top of everything else, this exercise is great for helping you get in shape for skiing, since the stretching movement in the calves is very similar to the one that takes place on skis.

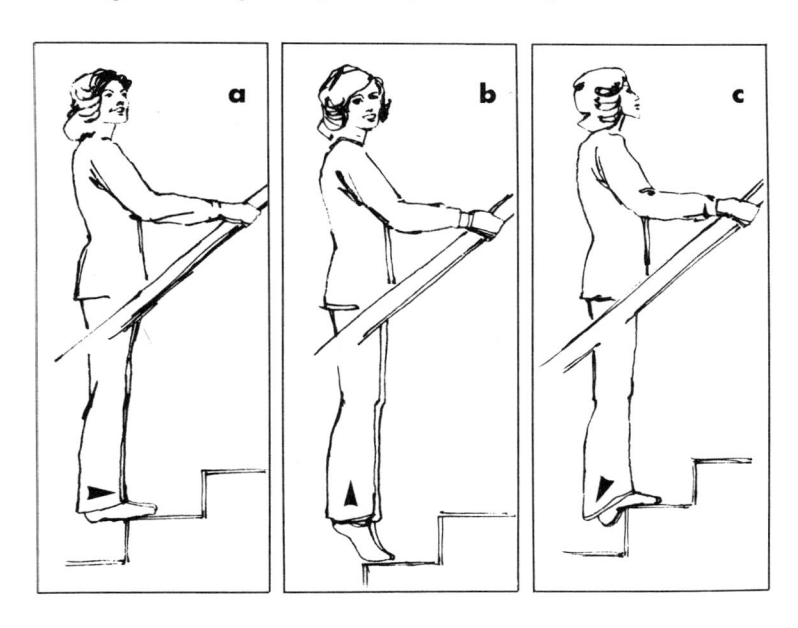

The amazing thing is that an exercise that does all these great things for you requires no special equipment and is simple to perform. All you do is find yourself a step, preferably one with a rail or wall next to it to hold onto. Stand with your toes on the edge of the step with your heels hanging out in space. Rise up high on your toes. Then, keeping your knees straight, sink way down, lowering your heels below the level of the step. You should feel a strong stretching in your calf muscles.

Dick does fifty of these with his toes pointed straight forward, fifty pigeon-toed, and another fifty with his toes pointed outward. He rests between each set of fifty. Dick says you should do these up to the point that you can't do one more. At that time you'll feel a chill of exhaustion run through your entire body. So far the best we've managed is twenty per position before reaching the exhaustion level. You needn't feel discouraged if you have to start off with ten or five or even three. The important thing is just to get started and work your way up gradually.

After you've done the Buerger-Allens for a spell and managed to recondition your feet and legs with the Bernsteins, you're ready to launch into Dave's CRIPE program and—who knows?—maybe tomorrow the Senior Olympics.

TIME ON YOUR FEET

The greatest problem maturity-onset diabetics have when it comes to sports and exercise is the fact that they're mature. Mature people do the greatest share of the world's work and they bear the greatest weight of the world's responsibilities. They are, consequently, the busiest and tiredest of people. As a result they often feel they are too busy and too tired for sports and exercise. Beware! As Dr. Tenley Albright, (nondiabetic) former Olympic figure-skating champion, cautions, "Just when

A Mature Attitude

you think you're too busy for sports [activity] is when you need it the most. When you're fit, you need less sleep and think more clearly. [Exercise] actually gives you more hours a day." For a diabetic, we might add, it can also give you more days in a lifetime.

A very busy thirty-eight-year-old professional photographer and mother we know of does gymnastic workouts at least three or four days a week. She even has an exercise mat at home so she can practice headstands and tumbling on days when her photography work makes it impossible to fit in a trip to the gym.

She firmly believes that "exercise is the best two-hour nap anyone can get, especially those diabetics like myself with large swings in blood sugar, who can actually feel the lethargy that a high blood sugar rests upon them. There is nothing that rejuvenates and negates that drag more rapidly and effectively than sport."

So you see you can't be too busy to exercise. Even Mary Tyler Moore, one of our favorite diabetic athletes-plus (and that's a big plus!) who has to have more demands on her time than you or we or all of us put together, still manages to fit a dance lesson into her lunch hour. Then there's Dan Rowan. Despite an overwhelmingly heavy schedule of performing and travel, he is able to find time for a daily extensive and intensive total body-building calisthenics program (twice a week with a professional instructor), for tennis practice or games four to six times a week, for participation in almost all the major celebrity tournaments (with a sizable number of wins notched on his racket), and even for sailing on his boat—sometimes as far as Hawaii.

Maybe it will help if you don't think of sports and

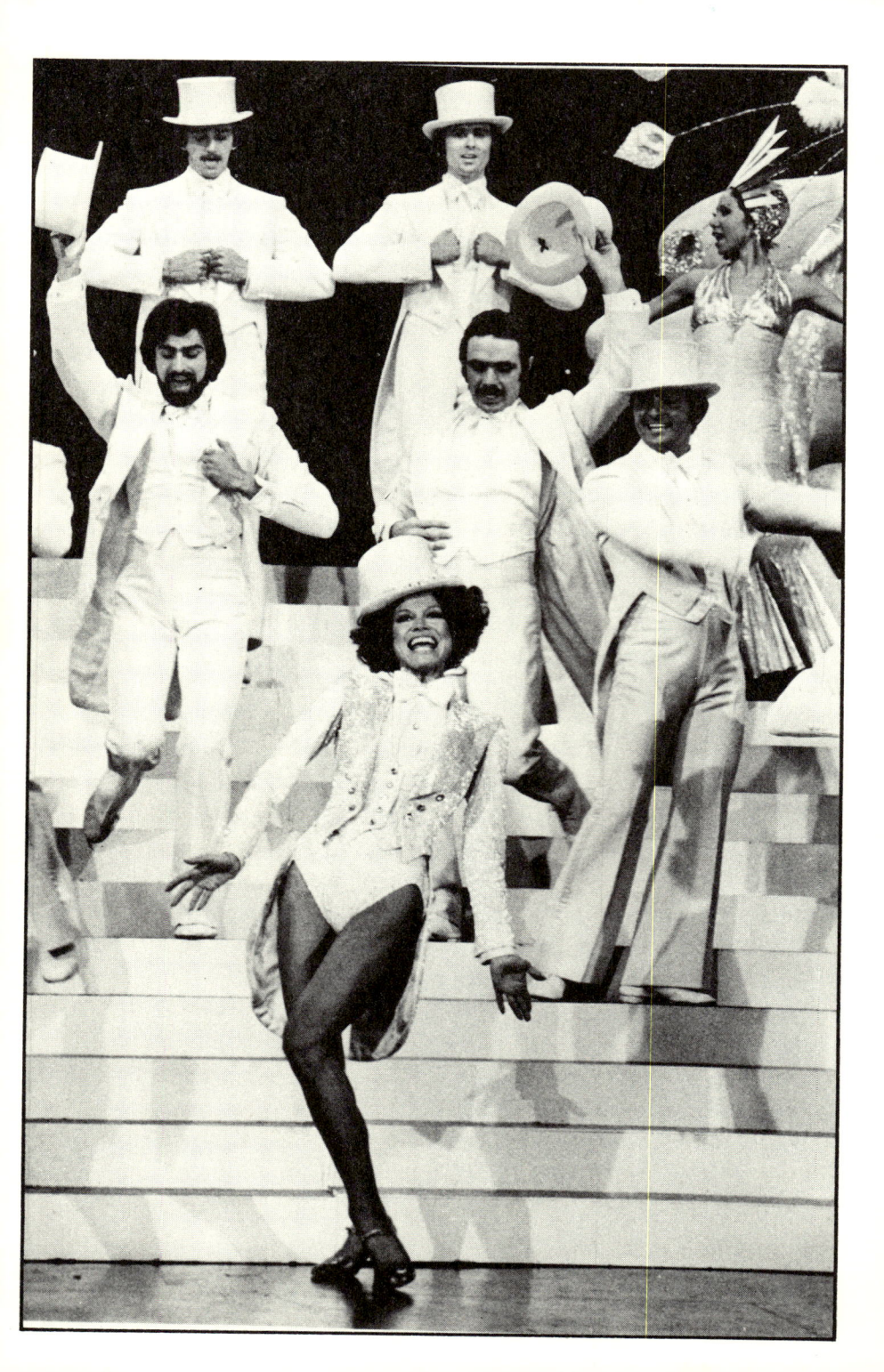

Mary Tyler Moore (left) in her TV special demonstrates the results of her daily dance lessons and her meticulous diabetes control. (Photo: Gene Stein, CBS)

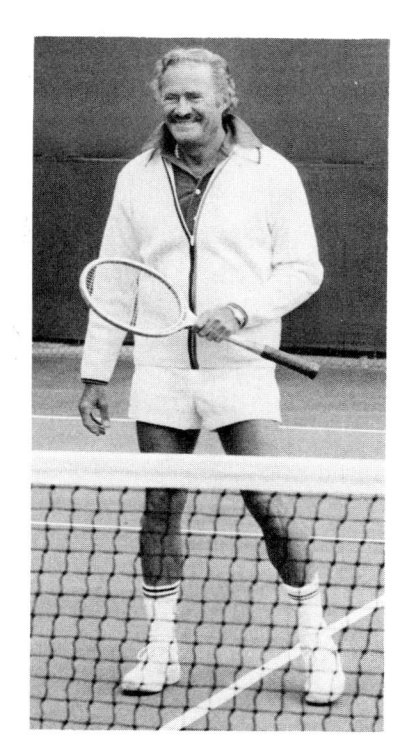

Dan Rowan (right) takes his sports and his diabetes seriously. (Photo: Frank Carroll, NBC)

exercise as fun (even though they are) but as a vital part of your diabetes treatment. In that way you won't feel it's wrong to take time away from work to exercise, but will instead feel it's wrong if you don't. This is called putting a twist on the Puritan ethic to make it work for your health.

5

Significant Others

Most of this book is designed to help and encourage you diabetics in the pursuit of exercise and sports. This section, however, is aimed at other people in your life—your parents, your doctors, and your coaches. These significant others sometimes have certain misconceptions and misunderstandings when it comes to dealing with you as a sports-minded diabetic. Since their problems frequently become your problems, we here offer some suggestions and possible solutions gleaned from remarks made by other diabetics and from our own experience in talking with mothers and fathers, with M.D.s, and with coaches and physical education instructors.

If any of this information seems applicable to your mother or doctor or coach, you could pass it on. It may help all of you as you work out your problems together. When dealing with these significant people in your life, however, we hope you—the diabetic—will hold one thing in mind: when they try to keep you on a short leash, they're acting out of the best of motivations—an excessive concern for your welfare. It's not easy to get mad at them for that. It's *possible*, mind you, but not easy!

MOTHER—M IS FOR THE MANY THINGS SHE WORRIES ABOUT

In our contact with diabetic kids who are involved in sports, a recurrent theme emerges:

"My parents were my only problem—worry, worry, worry."

"Mother's attitude was skeptical and I really had to prove myself to her. Father's attitude was good."

"My parents also encouraged me, but my mother always worried about me getting hurt."

"I have never had any fear from diabetes during sports. However, my mother constantly worries about me."

"Dad wanted me to play as soon as I was ready. But Mom always babied me."

"Some of my sports made my mother nervous."

"My mom was just plain motherly!"

Bill Talbert, too, had fretful parents when he started playing competitive tennis at age fourteen. "My parents gave me their support," he says, "but they were still nervous. My mother worried that I would fall over on the court, and my father smoked a pack and a half of cigarettes every hour I played."

Although there are a few overconcerned fathers (like Bill Talbert's chain smoker), we found Dad usually comes off as the good guy, while Mom is shown as fussbudgeting around and bugging the kid about being careful. In our experience, parents usually mutually overcompensate on every issue in the family—if one is overtense, the other opts for total relaxation—and those extremes could just as well be reversed between Mom and Dad. The parent who is home daily—and that's usually Mom, although even that situation is changing—feels the major burden of responsibility and hence adopts the tense role more often than not.

We're not going to be so unrealistic as to try to laugh off a mother's (or father's) worries. They exist. They're real. They're even justified. A mother worries about a child in sports, even if the child has no known physical problems. The Great Complicator, diabetes, complicates and compounds a mother's worries. The mother of a normal child worries about the major injury. The mother of a diabetic worries about the major injury but she also worries about the minor one—even a small cut or blister. How long will it take to heal? Will there be an infection? Blood poisoning? At the slightest scratch some mothers have visions of gangrene and amputation.

And how about insulin reactions? The mental image is always there in the back of the maternal mind. Her white-lipped child passes out cold or, even worse, is convulsing in the throes of shock. Unrealistic and unlikely? Sure. But the grim images remain.

Accentuate the Positive. As an old TV commercial put it, "What's a mother to do?" The way we see it, she has basically two approaches open to her—the negative and the positive. The negative approach is to do everything she can to keep her child out of any sports activity that involves any risk at all. This, of course, means out of any sport, period. If she succeeds in this, she can turn her child into a physical and mental and emotional invalid, into a skin-covered package of fears, into that "handicapped person" that all active and enthusiastic diabetics insist they're not. And indeed they are not. If a mother wraps her child in cotton batting and keeps him or her indoors, as we see it, what she is doing is not only negative, it is essentially destructive to what she values most, her child's health, because, as we keep repeating over and over again, exercise is a crucial part of diabetic therapy.

If, despite Mother's body check, the child is determined and manages to get into some sports, anyway, she can then drive child, coach, other family members, and herself crazy with her fears. She can impose so many restrictions that all joy is removed from the sport. The mother of a young rodeo rider went through such a period of excessive fear and concern after a scary insulin reaction. "For a long time every time he even turned over at night, I rushed to his room. Soon I realized I was making a nervous wreck out of all of us. And that I had to learn all I could, be prepared at all times, and put my trust in God." That philosophy of acceptance speaks loud and clear for all mothers.

Now, the other approach open to mothers—the positive one—is not the exact opposite of the negative one. It is not complete laissez-faire. It is not permitting children to do any damn fool thing that passes across their immature and inexperienced minds. This is just as unrealistic and potentially damaging as the negative approach. In dealing with a diabetic child, just as with a nondiabetic child, a mother has to sometimes put her foot down and put it down hard.

Our Maryland linebacker can see, in hindsight, the wisdom of his mother's firmness with him. "Former Notre Dame football star Coley O'Brien said I would need orange juice during the practices and the games, and I really did. I took it to the field and at first I would not drink it because the other guys weren't allowed to have

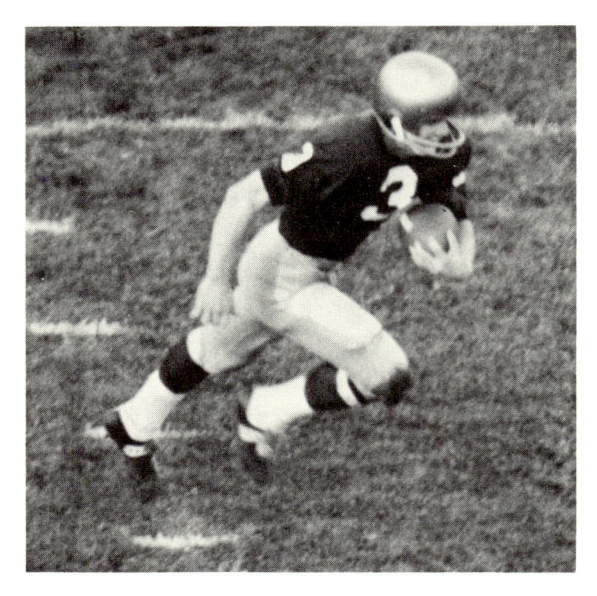

Coley O'Brien was a formidable football opponent and is a formidable friend to young diabetics who seek his advice on sports. (Photo: South Bend News)

anything and I didn't want any special privileges, but the coaches soon convinced me this was wrong, and my mom said I either drink the juice or not play. It was as simple as that, she said. I realize now how foolish it was of me, but I was a new diabetic and I guess I didn't want to feel different, but now I realize I am and there is nothing I can really do about it."

A good touchstone to go by is, "Would I let my child do this if he or she were not diabetic?" The parents of a young diabetic friend of ours have ruled out eighth-grade football for him. He doesn't feel bad about it, because his nondiabetic brothers have not been allowed to play the game, either. Football is just not that family's thing. Wrestling is—and that is a sport another diabetic gave up, because "my doctor told me not to wrestle because of the weight loss usually required. But that was fine with me because I hated wrestling and had no desire to do so anyway." One family's track meet is another family's poison, and that's OK. The only time you have to start worrying is when you find there are more poisonous activities than life-giving ones.

The Informer. The positive approach for mothers also involves converting energy that might be lost in worry and fret into some beneficial action on behalf of their child. For example, the mother of a diabetic daughter has prepared this letter, which she sends to summer camp personnel along with a roll of emergency Life Savers:

To All Camp Personnel:
Betsy will be able to participate in all regular camp activities, but a certain amount of observation and care should be exercised.

Diabetics are susceptible to shock. Betsy recognizes the first symptoms and immediately eats the Life Savers she carries, but should she miss the first symptoms, she may need your help. She will become very drowsy and later disoriented in speech and actions. At this point we will need you to *insist* she eat some candy (about a roll of Life Savers), or a high-sugar drink (Coke or orange juice) if she cannot chew. It will take five to thirty minutes for her to return to normal.

If she goes fully into shock and cannot take food by mouth, then contact the doctor, who has the proper medication for her.

Betsy has never gone beyond the first signs of shock where she eats the candy at her own instigation, but we feel you should be informed of what to do. We would also appreciate it if you would carry some of the Life Savers we have sent to camp with you when Betsy is in one of your classes.

This mother has another version of this letter which she gives to her child's teachers. She also sends both camp personnel and teachers a copy of the American Diabetes Association's information card, "What School Personnel Should Know About the Student with Diabetes." This card is reprinted in Appendix G, and you can either make photocopies of this reprint or write for copies at 25 cents each from:

> The American Diabetes Association
> 1 West 48th Street
> New York, N.Y. 10020

Another good service mothers can render for schools is to get together the funds to rent or buy the twenty-minute color film *Low Blood Sugar Emergencies in the Diabetic Child*. This film was produced cooperatively by a major school system and a county health department and is available from:

Lewis A. Rhodes
Juvenile Diabetes Foundation
Greater Washington Area
814 Lamberton Drive, Silver Spring, Maryland 20902

We previewed this film and found that it communicates a good understanding of diabetes in general and very specific information on the causes of low-blood-sugar emergencies, how to deal with them, and how to prevent them. The film is equally useful for educating coaches, camp counselors, scout and youth group leaders, and even parents of new diabetics.

Camp Crafty. How about those special diabetes summer camps for diabetic children? This is another area in which a mother can take positive action. She can become as investigative as Hercule Poirot to see what kind of reputation the diabetes camp in her vicinity has. (For the latest list of camps, write to the American Diabetes Association.) After grilling numerous diabetics and their parents and reading a lot about camps, we frankly cannot give them either wholehearted endorsement or flat condemnation. The reactions range from the vicious to the sublime:

"I spent two summers at a camp for diabetics when I first became diabetic. The only possible way that it might have helped me that I can think of was that I was so offended by the special clinical atmosphere of the camp and so offended by the special treatment demanded by some of the other campers because of their diabetes that I'm especially unwilling to let my diabetes prevent me from doing anything."

"My son attended diabetic camp last summer. It was a disaster for him and I don't believe he will go again. . . . The day we took him to camp we had to fill out a form stating how much insulin he was on, which was 16 units NPH and 8 units regular, yet the form we got back when he arrived home stated he arrived there on 12 units NPH and 6 units regular, which was wrong. They had also lowered his insulin, which I can understand with all the activities they have there, but to have him on only 4 units NPH was a bit much. It had taken us a year to put ten pounds on him, as he was only 57 pounds when we discovered he had diabetes. During his two-week stay at camp, he had lost five of them. His sugar level when he arrived home was very high. He had ketones, something he has never had at home. They had doctors, nurses, the whole bit there. I cannot understand why any child should return home in this shape."

Incidentally, this is not a supercautious, overprotective mother talking. Later she let her son go on a week's camping trip with his class. To take care of over sixty kids there was only one nurse. "He had a ball and did fine other than a fishhook in his finger."

Yet, on the other hand, we heard statements like:

"I attended Camp NYDA [New York Diabetes Association] for six years and learned that if my diabetes is properly controlled it won't be an obstacle to me."

"Camp Needlepoint, Hudson, Wisconsin . . . is where the different kinds of insulin were introduced to me. It was there where I learned about regular insulin. They also showed me different places for injections and how to give the shot there, the importance of amount of food and exercise. I guess it also made me aware of how many others have diabetes."

"As a child I attended a camp for diabetic children called Camp Whitaker. That camp experience attempted to instill into diabetic kids the principle that they're responsible for their own actions, safety, and enjoyment of life. In a matter-of-fact way the doctor in charge conveyed the assurance that diabetes was a problem which had rational means of control within the grasp of the diabetic himself."

Maureen Farrell, who received her nursing degree in 1975, wrote an encomium to her diabetes camping experiences in *Diabetes Forecast:*

> The eleven best summers of my life have been those spent at Camp Needlepoint, a summer camp for

young people with diabetes.... From everyday experiences I learned the relationships of insulin, diet and exercise instead of these just being entities that Mom always seemed to worry about when I was at home. Living with other diabetic children helped me to realize that I was not really so different from the rest of the world and still I was a unique individual....

Every year in returning to camp I learned new things about diabetes, besides thoroughly enjoying the camping experience.... A new environment with people who can really understand and empathize and share their experiences with diabetes has been really helpful. The opportunities for such sharing seldom exist in the child's home and school environment. I believe kids leave camp with an enriched understanding of themselves as people with diabetes. It helps to remotivate them for living with diabetes, adjust their own or adapt better attitudes toward life and glean pleasure and encouragement....

If attending a diabetic camp is half as rewarding for all campers and affects their lives and thoughts as much as it has mine, then diabetes camps are priceless.

The only general principle that bubbled forth out of the morass of conflicting statements on summer camps was that, on the whole, they're best for the newly diagnosed diabetic child. This is the one who needs help with the care and management of the disease. Many new diabetics first learn to give their own injections in camp under the influence of peer encouragement and pressure. The newly diagnosed diabetic may also need the reassurance that he or she is not the only one in the world with the problem, that there are lots more active, enthusiastic, likable kids who have it and are coping with it and leading happy lives.

Oddly enough, though, while diabetes camp can make children who feel abnormal feel more normal, it may have the reverse effect on children who have made the adjustment, who are used to taking care of themselves, and who spend most of their time on an equal footing with nondiabetics. Children like this can be irritated or disturbed at the constant harping on the diabetic condition and dislike the idea of being herded together with other diabetics as if they were an aberrant group.

Because of all these factors, the mother has to be not only a detective but a psychologist. She has to be able to determine, first, if her child is emotionally ready for the camping experience and, second, if a special diabetes camp would be better than a regular camp.

Finally, for a mother who worries about her child's being away from home, Dr. Theodore Van Dellen's advice is: "Short separations are good for both the parents and the child. This may be especially important in a situation where the parents have had to be overprotective. . . . However, don't leave [your child] with the impression that you want to get him out of your hair."

See How They Grow. The most important positive action mothers can take is to learn everything they possibly can about diabetes in general and their child's diabetes in particular and to transmit as much of that knowledge as feasible to their diabetic child. Instead of always being there to tell the child what to do or not do, positive mothers teach their children how to handle themselves in a diabetic emergency or, better still, how to prevent such situations from occurring. Since diabetes is a do-it-yourself disease, the do-it-yourself kid is always the winner in more ways than one.

All the effort and psychic pain of cutting the cord are worth it to mothers when they see the independent, active, unafraid individual they have released on the world. The glow of pride comes through in many letters we've received from mothers who took the positive approach. Here are just a few excerpts:

"I have a son who was diagnosed as a diabetic at the age of ten. He is now thirteen years old. When we first heard the news, my husband and I were crushed. It took us longer to accept this than it did my son. Today I have deep admiration for his accomplishments. He started to play Little League baseball the year before he had diabetes. Naturally, we were worried at first that sports would be too much for him. We continued to let him play baseball and this summer he ended Little League as an All Star and was an All Star every season. He hopes someday to become a major league ballplayer. . . . This boy, in spite of his diabetes, is a talented athlete, not just because he's my son. He has determination and drive. I know he would not write about his activities and I felt it would help other parents and children to know that they can lead almost a normal life. He is an honor roll student and all his teachers cannot believe he has a problem. He just seems to excel in everything he does."

"I am Brent's mother and I would like to tell you something about him that he wouldn't tell about himself. Brent will graduate from high school in June, and in addition to his athletic activities, since he became diabetic, he has earned his Eagle Scout Award, been the junior class president, was a representative to Idaho Boys State, and is a straight-A student. He has been awarded two academic scholarships for next fall. Needless to say, we are very proud of him. His attitude toward his disease and the way he has taken care of himself are just great and as a result his health is excellent."

"I feel we've been real lucky to have a diabetic for our son. I think we've all put a greater value on life and it's made us more aware of just everything. . . . Vince tickles you the way he goes about a sport or hobby or whatever. He really wants it to turn out right. Vince doesn't feel he is handicapped at all. He's happy about life all the time."

The kids with positive parents are very positive in their appreciation, too. A former defensive lineman for Fairleigh Dickinson University pretty much sums it up. "My parents never stopped me from being an active youngster. They never said, 'Bruce, don't play or you might get hurt.' They treated me like a normal child, and for that I will be eternally grateful."

THE STRANGE CASE OF DR. JEKYLL
AND MR. HYDE

As you probably remember, Dr. Jekyll was a learned physician who recognized the good and evil in all people and tried to separate the two in himself. By means of a drug he was finally able to create a separate personality—Mr. Hyde—who absorbed all his evil instincts. When he was Dr. Jekyll he was all good; when he was Mr. Hyde he was all evil.

We have noticed a similar phenomenon with diabetics' doctors. To hear the diabetics tell it, when it comes to encouraging them to lead normal, active, unrestricted lives, there is no middle ground. Their doctors are either all good or all evil.

First, let's hear a few words of praise for the Dr. Jekylls:

"My doctor is terrific. . . . He has always had an exceptional attitude about sports, both for diabetics and everyone. He's very athletic himself and advocates it for everyone. . . . I believe for any diabetic it is important to find such a doctor. Believe me, all doctors are not the same. My doctor has always tried different things on me as an individual and I'll be forever grateful to him."

"My doctor was just as enthusiastic as I was for me to get into sports. He taught me how to regulate my insulin dosage accordingly and felt that it was important for me to get exercise. He helped prepare me for the unexpected, i.e., insulin reactions. Therefore, he gave me the incentive to participate in sports and he gave me a relaxed attitude in coping with any adjustments I would need to make in my insulin dosage and diet in order to keep the diabetes under control."

"The doctor I have now thinks it's dynamite that I am as active as I am."

"Among the first questions I asked my doctor after finding that I had diabetes was whether I would have to restrict my activities. The one bright spot on that otherwise gloomy day was his reply that I shouldn't stop doing *anything* that I was doing or planned to do. His only reservation came when I asked about mountain climbing —he was a little doubtful about the wisdom of technical rock climbing: how could one reach a snack while clinging with both hands and feet to a rock face, should one suddenly become hypoglycemic. Since we hadn't done any roped climbing for years and weren't likely to be doing any very serious rock climbing, I was delighted with his enthusiasm for all other active sports, including mountain climbing."

" 'Don't be afraid to live, don't be an invalid, go out and ski and have reactions, tell the people what is going on, what to do—but don't be afraid—and have a good time.' That's what my good doctor said and that's what I'm doing."

Physician, Exercise Thyself. One of the best indications of whether a doctor will be an encourager of exercise or a discourager is whether he or she is an active sportsperson. If you go to a physically active doctor and ask about sports for diabetics, you're almost certain to get the kind of answer you want to hear.

When June's diabetes was first diagnosed in 1967 and she was unsure about whether or not it would be OK to take up skiing, she didn't consult someone like Phlegm J. Lethargic, M.D. Oh, no, she asked Dr. Merritt Stiles, former president of the U.S. Ski Association and second vice-president of the U.S. Olympic Committee, a man who, in his sixties, skied three or four days a week from November to April. It's not difficult to imagine the answer *he* gave.

Other diabetics report similar satisfactory results in their consultations with sports-minded physicians. "My doctor skis regularly," says one diabetic, "and he encourages participation in sports activities of any kind." An avid fisherwoman says, "My doctor is also a fisherman and that would not be the sport he would ban. Hopscotch—maybe."

Her point about doctors not forbidding their favorite sport was also noticed by a fourteen-year-old who wryly remarks, "One doctor I have right now is against wrestling because of the injuries he sees. But he took his six children to Montana twice this winter skiing."

And yet skiing isn't universally approved, either. "My doctor and I really don't see eye to eye on my skiing," says one skiing enthusiast in her forties. "He thinks it's a dangerous sport, anyway, and a diabetic skier is hard for him to comprehend. I know he visualizes me schussing the mountain and would not believe my snowplow if he saw it."

Most doctors, fortunately, are Dr. Jekylls. And a good thing, too, since diabetics who love the active life are usually strong willed and determined to (snow and otherwise) plow on, no matter what. As one such diabetic explains, "Rather than soliciting my physician's attitude, I told him that I simply was going to do everything that I wanted to in sports and that in my opinion the fact that I have diabetes is irrelevant. I think he is pleased with my approach to the problem."

A young female hockey player we know of has a similar idea. "My doctor just said I could participate in any activity I wished. I think I would have joined the team even if my doctor warned me not to. I think I know my capabilities more than anyone else."

And a handball enthusiast concurs. "My doctors and my family couldn't stop me from participating in sports; anyway, they go along with moderation."

For the final word on this subject we have our football "animal": "When I was in the hospital they all said no football but I just yessed them to death. Call it stubbornness or call it pride. I call it love of life."

Hyde Bound. There were diabetics, though, who gave us a negative picture of their doctors. A few of the complaints were petty irritations. We regularly heard diabetics grumble about overweight, chain-smoking doctors who had a don't-do-as-I-do-do-as-I-say philosophy. One disgusted diabetic stopped going to the meetings of his local diabetes association because, as he said, "I couldn't stand to sit there and be harangued about sticking to my diet by the medical advisor, who was so fat he wheezed when he climbed up onto the platform."

However, some of the complaints diabetics had about their doctors were deadly serious. The most common negative that diabetics voiced was when, like Mr. Hyde in full fang, the doctor would literally terrify them. This most often happened with a grim scare announcement of the diagnosis of the disease. The doctor who diagnosed June's diabetes was one of these fear merchants. "Everything about your life is going to have to change," he said, dealing out the exchange list diet as he launched into a catechism of the negative religion of diabetes.

And remember Dave Engerbretson's story of his doctor's "Things are going to be different. . . . You're going to have to slow down now." Dave admitted that this was said to him by a very old family doctor who had probably been treating patients since back in the days when diabetics were thought to have to coddle themselves—just as postoperative patients you now see trotting the corridors of the hospital the day after surgery were kept immobile for weeks.

The age of the physician, however, usually has little to do with it. Some of the most forward-looking physicians we know are in their sixties, seventies, and, believe it or not, eighties. We don't know the age of the doctor in the following story, but we do know that, even if you should seek, you couldn't find more of a Mr. Hyde than he:

"When our son was twelve we went to a new M.D., who on the first visit had to have a blood sugar run. He then came to talk to us. He told me and my son that if this boy doesn't change what he is doing about his illness, he'll be blind at eighteen, an amputee by twenty-one, and have kidney failure and be dead by forty. He wanted us to measure his insulin (which we always did), measure his food, take urine specimens at least three times a day, and measure his activity accordingly. He gave us a very grave outlook.

"We went along with this routine about two months. We left that doctor and I can honestly say I'm sure we'd not have our boy with us today if we'd kept up his idea for six months. In the time he was a patient there he was continually in a reaction. Very poor control with upset emotions. On each visit the doctor would repeat his bleak outlook for a normal life."

Needless to say, they changed doctors and "have had only encouragement since." Now, two years later, this young diabetic does weight lifting, plays basketball, skis (both water and snow), swims, hunts, rides a motorcycle, and participates in rodeos. According to his mother, he is "one of the healthiest kids around. Much healthier than our girls (older than he is)."

Shelly Lowenkopf believes that somebody has to educate these fear-merchant doctors. He says, "I think it vitally important that doctors be shown the extensive values of sports for diabetics so they will stop scaring the hell out of them with dire tales of athlete's foot developing into amputations, of broken bones resulting in casts being worn interminably, of the need to 'slow down and take it easy,' etc. There is an important difference between being a hypochondriac and an informed diabetic."

In defense of the ultracautious medical approach, we admit that most of the time the doctors are only showing their extreme concern for the diabetic's health. Still, a few doctors do have what seems to be a Procrustean approach to diabetes treatment. Procrustes, as you may recall, was the figure in mythology who had a bed for his guests. If a guest was too long for the bed, he chopped off the appropriate number of inches from the guest's legs to make him fit. If the guest wasn't long enough, Procrustes would stretch him to size. Thus it is with doctors who try to adapt a diabetic to their textbook treatment rather than to adjust the treatment to the individual diabetic. As one woman put it, "The most important thing for any sports-minded diabetic is to get a doctor who will treat you as an individual and not like one of a herd."

Some diabetics who discovered through experience that their doctor's set diabetes formula didn't work for them were hesitant to mention this to the doctor. Thom Underwood, as always, lays it on the line: "Hey, at one time I had a G.P. who told me a couple of Life Savers would pull you out of shock. I lied to him for a while about having to hit about five to ten cubes instead of Life Savers. That cat never went into insulin shock. Keep that in mind."

Of course, it isn't easy, not easy at all, for a doctor to figure out a personalized regimen for every diabetic. Look at it this way: You have only one diabetic to think about —yourself—and even for you, right there inside your own skin, feeling every sensation, it isn't easy to keep your blood sugar in the normal range. What works one day doesn't work the next. How can a doctor who sees you only every couple of months possibly predict all diabetic happenings and minutely adjust the treatment? Obviously, this is impossible. The doctor must, as one gymnast says, "place the diabetic responsibilities where they belong—on me."

This in turn means doctors must be willing to relinquish their total authority for diabetes care and become guides who can work *with* diabetics. They cannot be dictators of rigid policy. Not all doctors have the time—and this kind of cooperative treatment does take more time—or the flexibility to do this. And not all diabetics are willing and able and educated enough on the subject of diabetes to take on this much responsibility.

Many things conspire against independent action on the part of the diabetic. Books keep emphasizing that you shouldn't do thus or so without first checking with your doctor. Authors, including us, are always afraid that they'll be accused of usurping the doctors' prerogatives and trying to practice medicine without a license. We also quite genuinely fear that, heeding our advice to be independent, a diabetic may take some kind of independent goofy action and seriously undermine his or her health. And so over and over you hear: "Never begin an exercise program unless you check with your doctor," or "If you run ketones in your urine, check with your doctor," or "If you develop any kind of infection, be sure to check immediately with your doctor." We even read on a can of low-calorie but not sugar-free fruit that a diabetic should check with the doctor before eating it. It gets to the point that diabetics begin to feel that they shouldn't go to the bathroom without first checking with their doctor. And doctors must get to the point that *they* can't go to the bathroom without being interrupted by some diabetic who is trying to "check with the doctor."

Another problem comes from the fact that diabetics are not the world's easiest patients to deal with. One doctor told us he had a patient who had a leg amputated and was going blind and *still* refused to admit that he had diabetes. Diabetics also sometimes don't play it completely straight with their doctors. Some who are lax about their control shape themselves up with meticulous adherence to the diet when they know they're going in for a blood sugar. Diabetics have actually developed a reputation among doctors for being particularly stubborn and perverse. Some doctors won't even treat them. Apparently myths have developed concerning diabetics' behavior and even their basic nature. Here's something we read in *The Nutrition Handbook* by Carlton Fredericks. (This made June furious enough to raise her blood sugar by 20 points.)

> Hysterical traits are common among diabetics—some of them are actually on the borderline of mental disturbance. These patients are distant and reserved, wavering between feeble efforts at friendliness and suspicious reticence. They are tense, inhibited, yet somewhat childlike. For instance, they have little self-reliance, and when they talk about their feelings and personal problems there is a peculiar vagueness and a great deal of contradiction in their statements. The diabetic gives the impression of great internal activity, exhausting most of his available energy. Perhaps the major characteristic is indecisiveness. The

patient's initial reaction to illness is one of helplessness, although this is sometimes combined with self-blame.

Prescription for a Doctor. With all the built-in problems, what's the answer to the doctor-patient question for a diabetic who wants to lead an active life? Well, it's like the answer to the high/low blood-sugar swing. There's no one answer that's right yesterday, today, and tomorrow. You teeter along the line trying to strike the right balance.

Three firm suggestions we've come up with from our own experience and from the experience of diabetics we've talked to are these:

1. *Try to find a doctor who's a specialist in diabetes.* To quote one of the diabetics who feel very strongly about this:

"I think I've learned most about diabetes from the doctors I've had. Both of these doctors have been specialists. I think this is a sore point with me. I've met other diabetics who have been dealt with by a general practitioner. In most instances I find general practitioners don't know enough about diabetes and the controls and complications of diabetes and therefore the people I have met have had complications because they don't understand the situation. . . .

"G.P.s I have had contact with generally don't know as much as I know now about diabetes. This may sound funny, but you could see them expressing ideas which weren't really the truth or could lead a person to believe what he's doing is correct . . . when really the doctor didn't understand, as a specialist would."

This is no surprise—nor is it a reflection on the G.P.; he couldn't possibly be expected to understand as much as a specialist who sees diabetics all day long every day. The specialist knows not just the theme of diabetes but the myriad variations on that theme as well. As a consequence, specialists are generally more flexible in their treatment and allow their patients more latitude, something a diabetic wants and needs in order to lead that normal life you always hear about.

Where and how can you find a specialist? If your local library has a copy of the *Directory of Medical Specialists*, you can use that, but it takes quite a bit of detective work. You have to first look up the internal medicine specialists in your area, then see which ones have something about diabetes in their experience (for example, past president of the local diabetes association). You can also call a good hospital and ask who on their staff is a diabetologist. Another technique is to get in touch with your local diabetes association and ask for their recommendations.

Naturally, it is always possible to run up against specialists who are so diabetes oriented that they can't see the patient for the disease, can't treat the person as a total human being, are more interested in their lab work with mice than their office visits with people. Here you have to make your own evaluation of the treatment you're getting. If you're not happy with it and if you can't discuss the situation with your doctor and try to work things out, then we come to piece of advice No. 2.

2. *Don't be afraid to change doctors.* People, especially diabetic people, do it all the time. June had two doctors before she found happiness with a third. Diabetic after diabetic we've talked to count their doctors like rosary beads. Changing two or three times is not unusual,

especially when overprotective doctors are the problem. Of course we're not advocating that diabetics shop around until (if ever) they manage to find doctors who will go along with everything and anything they want to do. If that's what you're after, then why spend time and money going to *any* doctor?

No, find a doctor you can *respect*. Find one with whom you work well. A doctor-patient relationship is not a tug-of-war but a cooperative effort, more like a two-person rowing team with both of you working toward the same goals of good health, good control, and a good life.

3. *Always seek a second medical opinion* if your treatment is not working or if your doctor makes what you consider an unreasonable restriction. This point was brought home to us by a young woman bicycle enthusiast who got into trouble with a vaginal yeast infection and aggravated the condition by continuing to cycle. "I was told by my former gynecologist," she said, "that, as he put it, having sex once per week was too often for a diabetic woman or else she would have a yeast infection all the time." She sought another opinion and got one—and it was that the first doctor was mistaken. She offers this advice to other diabetics, based on her own doctor experiences:

    1. Get a second medical opinion if you are unhappy with your treatment.

    2. If an infection is on the rampage, make sure it gets stopped. Do not agree to merely take two aspirin, wait until tomorrow, and call the doctor again if it is still bothering you. One of the bad results, for women, of running sugar while an infection is rampaging can be a very nasty yeast infection.

    3. Don't take medicine if you have any reason to

suspect that you are allergic to it; discuss it with your doctor.

"*Discuss* it with your doctor." That's a small but very important change from "Check with your doctor." It implies an exchange of ideas, of working out diabetic problems together. That is the secret of how both physician and diabetic patient can be Dr. Jekylls. That is how to keep an evil Mr. Hyde from appearing anywhere in the consultation room.

FAINT-HEARTED MENTORS

The old sports edict of "It matters not if you win or lose but how you play the game" should be modified for diabetics to read, "It matters not if you win or lose but if you get to play the game." Diabetics aren't always given that chance. Strangely enough, there are coaches and P.E. teachers and recreation leaders—the very people whose goal is supposed to be to get *everyone* to participate—who try to keep diabetics out.

One high school girl, who in her out-of-school hours leads an extremely active sports life, encountered one of those coaches who try to slam the locker room door in the diabetic's face. The girl enrolled in the swimming class, but when the coach learned she was diabetic his instant reaction was, "Aha! Now what happens if you're in the pool and you're swimming and you have a reaction? You'll be drowned and we'll be sued."

The coach forthwith sentenced the girl to a class in "adaptive P.E." (that's a euphemism for sitting around doing nothing, because you're "too delicate" for the regular sports program). The girl fought the decision and appealed to the principal. To his credit, he overruled the coach's decision and admitted the girl to the swimming class. The result, she told us, was that it "made me swim extra hard the entire semester and I almost killed myself doing it."

It's bad enough for diabetics to feel they have to overprove themselves to a coach, but it's even worse when they feel they have to hide the fact of their diabetes from the coach. There are closet or, in this case, locker diabetics all across the country. We heard from several, who said things like:

"My last coach didn't even know I was a diabetic."

"When I was on the high-school ski team, the coach knew nothing about my diabetes."

"No, my soccer coach does not know I am a diabetic."

"If the sports instructor seems to be the type to put up a fight about my involvement, I simply forget to tell him I'm diabetic."

This sort of hiding of diabetes can result in some ludicrous situations:

"My sophomore year at college I was traveling on a bus to St. Louis, where we had a baseball game. It was the first game I was going to start as shortstop. My coach didn't know I was a diabetic and only a few players knew, so I hid in the back of the bus. I injected back there. Nobody ever knew."

But ludicrous situations are not the worst kind; dangerous ones are. There can be dangerous situations when a coach is not aware that a diabetic is on a team or in a class and is not aware what should be done if an emergency occurs.

How, then, are diabetics going to get around these

faint-hearted mentors? How are they going to get their chance to participate without having to pay for it with the risks of deception? A few diabetics try to prove themselves first, then tell:

"I perform first, then tell the coaches. Most coaches won't let you play because they think that you are not physically strong enough for the pain. If you produce, they will keep you."

This works pretty well if you're a hotshot athlete. A coach isn't going to bench the star center or pitcher or quarterback or sprinter, if it turns out after the first win or two that the person's a diabetic; that coach will manage to make whatever adjustments are necessary. But is this fair? (And sportspeople traditionally have fairness as their stock in trade.) Should diabetics have to be better than everyone else just to get the same chance? That's exactly the kind of treatment minorities and women have been complaining about—the fact that they have to be better than the next person to be considered as good.

Conversely, diabetics don't expect to make the team simply because they have diabetes. No one is asking that a team have its token diabetic or token epileptic or token asthmatic or token any other disease. All that's asked is that people who would make a team if they didn't have diabetes make it if they do.

As for P.E. classes and recreational outings, diabetics should *never* be excluded unless they refuse to acknowledge their diabetes and take the responsibility for its care. Happily, young sports-minded diabetics of this type are as rare as pecan pie on Bobby Clarke's training table.

Ignorance Is Blitzed. When it comes to coaches who exclude diabetics, we often have to "forgive them, for they know not what they do." Learning about the relationship of diabetes and exercise and the handling of diabetic problems is evidently not a universal part of the professional preparation of sports instructors. Over and over and over again we've heard the same story from diabetics:

"My coaches knew I had diabetes but their knowledge was usually rather vague."

"Coaches don't know much about diabetes."

"I was on a swim team in high school; my coach had practically no knowledge whatsoever of diabetes."

"The coaches I have played for have only a layman's general idea of what is involved with diabetes."

"I have never had a coach who had adequate knowledge of diabetes."

Clearly, forgiveness is not enough. Something else is required. Coaches are going to have to be coached on the subject of diabetes. Physical educators are going to have to be mentally educated and recreation leaders are going to have to be re-created into persons knowledgeable in diabetes care.

And who is going to do this? Who else but those who are most concerned, diabetics and their families? They will have to press reading material into the coaches' hands. Pamphlets on the subject are available free from the American Diabetes Association and its local affiliates. One particularly succinct and useful item is the ADA's information card, "What School Personnel Should Know About the Student with Diabetes" (see Appendix G). There are also many books on the subject. Modesty should forbid our mentioning our own *Diabetes Question and Answer Book*, but it doesn't, because it's the one book we know of that was written specifically for people who know nothing—or next to nothing—about diabetes. Since this is such a visual age, however, many mentors might prefer to absorb their information from the movie we mentioned earlier in this chapter, *Low Blood Sugar Emergencies in the Diabetic Child.*

After the coach has a basic foundation of diabetes information, the diabetic can discuss any individual peculiarities and any special needs. That's usually all it takes. Once coaches or P.E. teachers understand what diabetes is, know how it works, and how to head off the demon insulin reaction, they usually begin to see that it is, as Dave Engerbretson says, "No big deal."

Conscientious Objection. It is possible for a coach to become too conscientious, to try to take on too much responsibility for the diabetic. While this isn't as bad as refusing to have anything to do with a diabetic, it can cause problems.

When he speaks to coaches on the subject of diabetes, Dave Engerbretson always warns, "You have to remember that all aspects of diabetic control and treatment are the diabetic's own responsibility. They are certainly not yours. As a teacher and coach it's not up to you to chase this guy around and say, 'Well, did you have your insulin?' or 'You shouldn't eat this' or, if you see the guy with a 7-Up in his hand, 'Put that down! You're a diabetic!' If he gets out of control, has problems, that's *his* problem. It isn't yours."

One of Bobby Clarke's trainers, Frank Lewis, has the right idea. "We keep on hand a good supply of Coke and don't bother Bob at all about diabetes. He knows when he needs something sweet and he takes care of himself well."

P.E. teachers and coaches *can* bug diabetics unmercifully. This both drives them crazy and sets them apart from their classmates or teammates—something almost every diabetic cordially detests. One girl who had taught her diving coach how to administer glucagon in an emergency reported that the coach would follow her around "asking me if I felt all right and telling me if I felt an insulin reaction coming I should take care of it right away, because she hates giving injections."

It is not the coach's responsibility, either, to tell others about the diabetic's disease. To quote Dave again, "It's up to the diabetic if he wants people to know, and he's the one who ought to tell them. You shouldn't stand up some day when he's not around and make the announcement that Johnny is a diabetic and this and that and the other thing. It's not your place to do that, but at the same time I think the diabetic ought to do it."

Soft-Hearted Mentors. The other thing a coach can overdo is the sympathy and understanding bit. Some feel so sorry for a diabetic that they give special privileges to make up for the disease. This is quickly resented by other team or class members. It is also resented by most diabetics, because, again, they don't like to be made to feel different. There are a few—*very* few—who would take advantage of such a situation. There are fewer still who use their diabetes as a device to get their own way. As Dave explains it:

"While we're going to have to make certain allowances for the metabolic demands of the diabetic, I don't think you should let the diabetic take advantage of the situation and you shouldn't let him play on his needs to take advantage of you."

Dave experienced just such a virtuoso player one

summer when he was doing some fly-fishing workshops on a dude ranch in Montana. The ranch was for older children, and among those children was one diabetic. According to Dave, "That guy played his disease like a finely tuned violin."

If something came up that he didn't want to do, out would come the refrain, "Well, gosh, I'm a diabetic, so I'd better not take that ride" or eat that food or whatever. And then when there was something he *wanted* to do that they didn't want him to, the theme would be, "Well, you know I'm a diabetic and I need my exercise now, so you'd better let me take out that horse for a ride."

Any time he didn't get his way with another kid he'd start a fight, and after it was over you'd hear a *symphonie pathétique* on how his blood sugar was low or he would never have done such a thing. They finally had to refund the boy's money and ship him home because he was ruining the summer for everyone else—and he wasn't doing himself much good, either.

Paying Your Do's. Besides these general don't's for coaches and P.E. teachers, there are a few specific do's :

1. Do get an OK from the physician if a diabetic is going to be engaging in a rough, demanding, competitive sport like football, hockey, or wrestling.
2. Do let diabetics take care of their needs, such as stopping to eat, without making them feel as if they're a drag on the group.
3. Do learn how to administer glucagon, should a diabetic ever become unconscious in a reaction. (Check first to make sure your state has no laws against nonmedical personnel giving injections.)

4. Do always keep candy or soft drinks or juice or something on hand for emergency situations.

5. Do try to know each diabetic's personality well enough to tell, when tempers flare, if it's the personality or the low blood sugar that's popping off.

6. Do arrange a signal with diabetics so that if they're in the middle of a game and start to get a reaction they can give you the high sign and you can get them out and get something sweet into them.

Most of all, *do* keep your cool and *do* remember: "It's no big deal."

Stout-Hearted Mentors. Another mighty do for coaches and P.E. teachers is to emulate the really terrific stout-hearted mentors who realize that regular physical exercise is as important to a diabetic as insulin or diet and who don't just permit diabetics to participate but encourage them. With sports professionals like these in charge, the problems work themselves out very easily, as their students report:

"My coach has adequate knowledge of diabetes. (She read up on it after finding out I had it.) We work together to prevent problems."

"In football the assistant coach was also diabetic and this helped me a great deal. He was able to help the other coaches understand my problem. All of my coaches in high school in all sports have helped and encouraged me."

"I feel my coach is very knowledgeable as to diabetes. She makes sure I am OK and insists I tell her if I'm not. Any time I need food, etc., she says just to get it, no questions, nothing. And if I need help to just tell her. But she always treats me as one of the girls, not as a standout or someone special, but normal."

Some coaches go way beyond the call of duty—in fact, way out on a limb—for their diabetic athletes. This was the case with Theresa Harris's scuba-diving teacher. (You'll remember you last saw Theresa in a Smokey the Bear costume.) After an initial reluctance to let her participate, he—well, let's let Theresa tell it:

"My most prized accomplishment as a diabetic was receiving my scuba license. My instructor didn't seem to like the idea of a seventeen-year-old girl in his scuba class, but when he found out I was a diabetic, he really disagreed. I can be a very convincing person when I feel I have to, so after a half hour of talking with my instructor, he signed me up in his class. Of course, I got tested quite fully in the pool before our first ocean dive. When the Saturday of the dive came, I was so excited I forgot my insulin in the morning. I wasn't far from home when I remembered, so I turned around and went back home for my shot.

"In full gear (wet suit, regulator, tanks, weight belt, mask, and fins) I was ready for my test. The test consisted of backing through the breakwater and then swimming out to a boat waiting for us. Dennis, my instructor, took me alone so he could give me his undivided attention. I am proud to say I did just as well as anyone else.

"The day of my certification dive turned into a terrible experience. Dennis took my buddy partner and me out to do our qualifying dive. Everything was going well until we started to dive deep. I was diving with a cold and a 101-degree temperature, because this was the only day we were supposed to have in order to qualify. Down about ten feet my body suddenly became unequal. One of my ears popped, but the other refused to. This caused an immediate and very bad nosebleed.

"My mask filled up with blood and scared me half to death. I surfaced and ripped my mask off while Dennis inflated my life vest. Having to be carried out of the water and up a terribly steep cliff, I feared I would never dive again. Dennis and my buddy made a bed for me in the back of a station wagon to take me to the dive shop.

"I can't really explain what it is like to be unequal. It was just as if I had ten left legs and fourteen upside-down heads! At the dive shop Dennis gave me some pills to pop the other ear, though I didn't really feel better until the next day.

"Now, although my being unequal had nothing to do with diabetes—it can happen to anyone who dives—I was afraid they would use it as an excuse to keep me from ever getting my certificate. Can you believe the next week Dennis called me and asked if I wanted to try again at the end of the month? Like most fairy tales, this story has a happy ending. I did get my certificate, and if it wasn't for having such a beautiful person like Dennis as an instructor, I know my certificate would just be another dream."

6

Oh, the Disadvantages of Being a Diabetic— and (Believe It or Not) Oh, the Advantages

We would certainly blow our credibility with you if we tried to skip around smiling and claiming that there are no disadvantages to being a diabetic when it comes to sports endeavors. Just in case you haven't noticed any of these disadvantages, we'll point out a few.

FEAR OF FLYING

To begin with, there are a number of activities that are illegal for a diabetic. The restriction on flying an airplane is the one that particularly upsets several of the diabetics we talked to. As a freewheeling, free-spirited group, they hate the idea of not being able to experience the ultimate winging-off freedom. As one put it, "I wanted my pilot's license, but the government said that diabetics weren't allowed to take their pilot's license and this is an understandable situation. I don't really argue with them on it. However, it is the only thing that I would have liked to have done and have not been able to do."

All is not lost, though. There is a student at the University of California at San Diego who is living, flying proof that some diabetics do operate planes with a licensed pilot in the cockpit beside them. "For me, the sky's not the limit," he says, "I've been flying for as long as I can recall. F.A.A. rules prevent me from getting my private pilot's license. I hope someday to remedy this by getting a special restricted license. Until then, I satisfy myself by flying with another licensed pilot. They merely sit back and let me do the flying—it's perfectly legal. I fly both power planes and sailplanes. I am currently the safety officer and an active member of the University of California at San Diego Soaring Club.

"I should qualify what I said about getting a restricted pilot's license. I would like to receive one only for gliders, since I can see the validity of banning diabetics from piloting power planes. They could do a lot of damage in the event of some 'diabetic mishap.' However, it seems to me and a lot of other qualified people that a solo diabetic pilot flying a sailplane in a remote area could, at the worst, only hurt himself. I would like to stress that my view is that a diabetic person should only receive a restricted license for solo flying of gliders in remote areas, contingent upon a release from a physician that the diabetic is under good control. The diabetic pilot would be a person quite knowledgeable and aware of his or her condition, and a person who would take his diabetes into account while flying (for example: increasing the blood-sugar level slightly in order to reduce the chance of insulin shock). Presently the only kind of solo flying available to the diabetic is either hang gliding or illegally flying somewhere out in the desert."

Several diabetics believed that parachute jumping and skydiving are also sports that are prohibited to diabetics, but we checked with the F.A.A. and it's not true. We decided that those diabetics who had trouble just bumped up against some special restrictions of individual skydiving groups. Our theory was later confirmed by a thirty-two-year-old sky diver who told us about his first experience. "On the form that was required to be filled out the day we took the skydiving instructions, there was a statement asking if you had, among other diseases, diabetes. I told the instructor I did. He said I would have to have a doctor's permission before I could jump. I decided to take the training session that day anyway. By evening I was so excited about jumping that I pleaded with the instructor to let me do it. I told him I'd had diabetes for seventeen years and had never had any serious reactions. I guess I was pretty convincing—or lucky. I got to jump that day. Climbing out onto the step of the plane, one of the last things I would have thought about would have been having diabetes."

SCOUTS' DISHONOR

A couple of diabetic sportspeople experienced the disadvantage of being denied an opportunity to enter professional sports because of their disease. "When I played high school baseball," reports Joe Brink, "I was exceptionally good and was approached by professional scouts to play pro baseball. They refused to sign me because of my diabetes. It was one of the biggest disappointments of my life."

Another diabetic was scouted—and turned down—for pro hockey. Fortunately these thwartings took place several years back, and in the meantime there have been

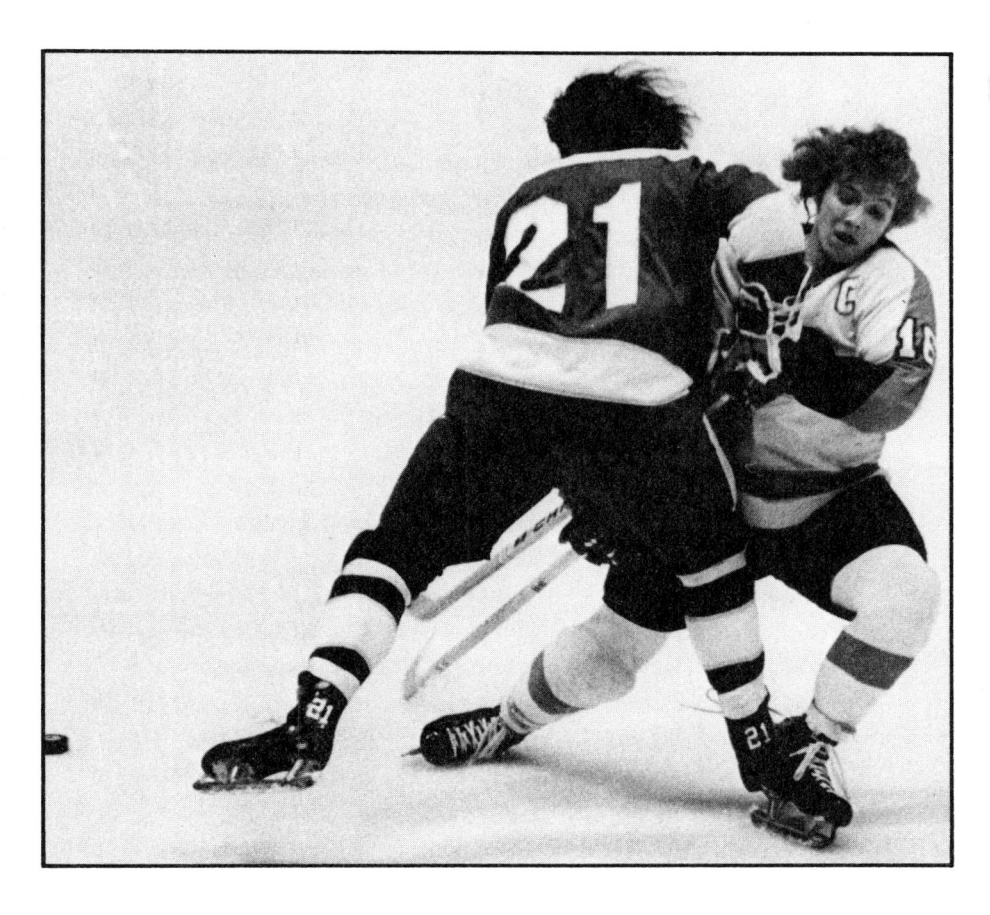

"The Iceman Cometh"—Bobby Clarke shows the world you can live like a diabetic and play like a champion. (Photo: Philadelphia Flyers)

enough successful diabetics in pro sports to change a few of the warped minds of the scouts.

What happened with Bobby Clarke no doubt contributed a great deal toward the dewarping process. In the player draft of 1969 sixteen players were chosen before Clarke. Finally, when it was the second time around for Philadelphia to choose, the Flyers' scout, Gerry Melnyk, urged the General Manager to take Bobby, predicting, "If he doesn't make your club immediately, he'll be called up by Christmas." The manager checked with a Philadelphia doctor about what problems diabetes might cause. Apparently he got the right answer, because the Philadelphia Flyers drafted Bobby Clarke.

Most of the sixteen players chosen before Bobby are unknowns today, while the man the other ten teams passed over because of his diabetes went on to become the National Hockey League's youngest captain and to win the most valuable player award and the Bill Masterson trophy for his qualities of perseverance, sportsmanship, and dedication to hockey. He became only the ninth person in history to score 100 points. He led his team to a Stanley Cup victory. And in the process of all this he became an acknowledged superstar.

If still another sports superstar, Jackie Robinson, had developed his diabetes a little earlier than he did, he might have done as much for breaking down the barriers for diabetics as he did for blacks.

But restrictions still remain in some areas. Thom Underwood was prevented from taking an Outward Bound course in wilderness survival. And Dave Engerbretson ran into trouble when he tried to get certified as a backpacking guide in New England:

"I went to leadership school and everything was going along swimmingly and all of a sudden somebody picked up on the fact that I was a diabetic. I hadn't tried to hide it from anybody, but apparently the leaders didn't know it. All of a sudden I got this phone call, 'Would you come out to so-and-so's house? We want to have a special session with you.' I went out and there were these people on the examination committee. (Fortunately one of them was a physician.) They had called me out to break the news to me that there was no way they were going to certify a diabetic as a guide. 'We can't have a diabetic going off into the mountains and being responsible for the lives of other people,' and so on.

"Well, we sat around for a few hours. I had a pretty good understanding and knowledge of what was going on, and I managed to convince them that I wasn't going to kill anybody and I knew enough about my own condition to handle it. The end result was that I *did* get certified. But they were right. They were right in making darned sure that I as a diabetic knew enough about the disease to handle an outdoor situation."

THE ENEMY WITHIN

But these are all external restrictions and problems for a diabetic. There are also the internal restrictions and problems—the mind and body happenings that cause a diabetic not to be able to do his best at a sport, or not to be able to do the sport when he wants to, or to have to stop doing it when he doesn't want to, or—well, let's hear it straight from the sources:

"I guess I have to admit, yes, diabetes does interfere

with my sport—sometimes consciously and sometimes unconsciously. I am scared that I'm going to start shaking, get a headache, become very hot and weak (reaction) and then I won't be able to compete or won't be able to finish the sport. I feel then that I'm letting the team down and myself, too, because after all the work put into it I want to be able to show something for it. This causes me . . . problems because sometimes I give a little less insulin or eat a little too much to insure myself against a reaction and then I get symptoms because of too much sugar. . . . Sometimes practice will be half done and I get a reaction and it takes me the other half to get back to normal and then practice is over. This makes me mad, because I have missed precious moments of practice or else sometimes I am checking sugar and I don't have much umph or energy at practice and I feel terrible but I suppose everybody—normal and diabetic—feels like this so I suppose some of these days are just my off days, too. But it upsets me and makes me want to work and try harder."

"In competitive golf situations there is probably an unfavorable impact on my concentration at times when I have to think about beating my diabetic opponent as well as par. When I should be thinking about swing mechanics and strategy, I may be worried about how I'm going to get from the ninth green to the snack bar and back to the tenth tee without interrupting play."

"In wrestling I cannot raise and lower my weight at will, as most wrestlers do."

"In high school, I wrestled and always tired out so easily. Didn't know how to regulate myself well then, though. In competitive sports such as Ping-Pong and tennis, I have been a little frustrated at times because there would be nothing I could do about a sudden low but take carbohydrates and wait for my energy level to climb."

"I borrowed a bike and tried the Century [100-mile ride] but had to quit after 90 miles. I ran out of high-carbohydrate food and didn't want to take any chances."

"The diabetes 'interferes' with my exercise or my participation in sports mainly in that I cannot exercise vigorously before a meal without having to consume gobs of sugar. . . . Another minor way that having diabetes interferes with my sports is that occasionally I have to stop what I'm doing to take sugar or eat some candy. . . . When I ski I must stop to eat lunch on time. Sometimes this is a little inconvenience."

"Backpacking for a period longer than a week requires enough food to the point that weight becomes a factor."

"Spur-of-the-moment decisions to go biking are usually passed up, if the hour for cycling is too close to mealtime. I would be afraid of bringing on an insulin reaction. While it would be nice to ski through the regular lunch hours of eleven to one when lift lines are short, I wish it were possible to avoid my diet's timing requirements. . . . Timing is also a problem when I take a week's vacation at a resort. . . . Vacation days usually start with tennis at seven and breakfast delayed until nine thirty. I usually eat fruit before the tennis time. With a late breakfast my friends bypass lunch and I delay my lunch until one or two which permits me to last until the vacation dinner hour of eight or eight thirty. Naturally, when friends have invited me to play tennis at a particular time, I either have to say no or see if a change in time is possible in case the planned hour is at a time when my blood sugar might be approaching a low point. More than anything I resent having to keep all my athletic endeavors within a limited amount. If I were to do any one of them to too great a degree, I would throw my whole system off balance."

"Limits my stamina, my length of excursion is from breakfast to lunch. I'm careful from eleven to twelve. It's kind of touchy then. Lunch to dinner I can't or let's say won't climb another mountain. Takes too much out of me, takes at least three days afterwards to get things back together."

"I think I haven't gotten over the psychological effects of it all yet. I sometimes feel inferior and that I can't play as well as before, so I don't. Tennis is a lot mental attitude, and that is where I have my problems and fears."

Achilles Heal. The first book June ever read about diabetes, *Diabetic Care in Pictures* by Helen and Joseph Rosenthal, had an entire chapter called "Skin Injuries and Infections from Skin Injuries." There were almost hysterical warnings about the consequences of such skin damage as hangnails, and cautions about the use of adhesive tape, which can break the sensitive diabetic skin when removed. All this was capped off with the cheerful tidings that if you did break your skin and the wound became infected, as it easily could, then the infection would throw your diabetes out of control and present you with a double problem. No, make that a triple problem, because gangrene seemed to always be in the wings waiting to put in its grisly appearance. June immediately felt she ought to move inside a bell jar and just sit there doing nothing.

Clearly the slow healing of injuries—or in some cases the *fear* of slow healing—can be a disadvantage for a diabetic who wants to participate in sports. But is this disadvantage necessary? No and yes. The official healing scoreboard for the diabetics who commented on it is: 17 said they healed less quickly than nondiabetics; 24 said they healed as quickly as nondiabetics; 4 even claimed to heal more quickly than nondiabetics, a claim which we feel should be taken with a grain of salt—or perhaps a grain of penicillin.

Reading between the lines and listening between the words, we came to the same conclusion about diabetic healing as did Dick Bernstein.

"I do find that when the diabetes is under good control," he says, "wounds, cuts, and the like heal rapidly. When it is under poor control they heal more slowly."

Dr. Olson is very specific on the subject of healing of injuries to diabetic sportspeople. "The well-controlled diabetic below the age of fifty ordinarily will heal as well, and with no more infection than one would encounter in the nondiabetic. However, over the age of fifty with the increased incidence of atheromatous changes in the arteries, the problem isn't as much due to diabetes as it is to the blood supply to the extremities. Even with meticulous control of blood sugar, if the blood supply to an injured extremity is poor, the patient is going to experience difficulty in healing and, indeed, in some cases, total healing becomes very difficult."

If it is true that a young in-control diabetic heals as well as his nondiabetic counterpart, why then are doctors so concerned? Why do diabetics say such things as the following?

"When it was first discovered that I was a diabetic, the doctor I had at the time advised me that I shouldn't ski or participate in other sports where I could get hurt."

"The doctor who set my arm about had a heart attack when I told him I was a diabetic."

"The complications I have are doctor feelings about me playing sports when an injury is brought to their attention. My brothers have had injuries of the same sort and never get the guff that I do. . . . Doctors spent a lot more time checking on me and charging my parents for the calls."

Dr. Olson makes it easy to understand why doctors are so seemingly overly concerned about injuries to a diabetic. It's because, he explains, "Although an in-control diabetic under fifty does heal as rapidly as a nondiabetic, well over 50 percent of the young diabetics never experience what we consider good control. If these young people are injured and have continued hyperglycemia, then they are going to have more problems."

And they're also going to have grim stories to tell, such as:

"Several years ago an opponent jumped on my left foot and I continued to play ball, and my diabetes got out of control. I continued to play with this bad foot until an abscess formed. I had to be hospitalized for four weeks. Now I am wiser and take better care. I watch out for injuries, especially of the feet. And I give these injuries constant and immediate attention by resting, soaking the injured part, and controlling the diabetes."

"I have ripped up my knees twice motorcycling. The first time I got a good infection due to the inadequate medical care I received at a local hospital. However, my doctor quickly took care of that problem. Healed quickly, are you kidding? I walked around like a penguin for one and a half months."

"I had a bad blister on my sole after running ten miles

at 95 degrees F. The blister broke and became infected with several pathogenic organisms. Slow to heal and cure (probably because I was diabetic)."

We get the message. Good control and meticulous care of injuries are vital unless a diabetic wants to carry a heavy disadvantage in his athletic equipment bag.

Muscling In. Some diabetics who want to get deeply involved in a sport where size and weight are assets consider that diabetes has kept them from progressing as they would have without diabetes. Dick Bernstein explains the why's of this: "I notice that juvenile-onset diabetics are almost inevitably quite slim.... When the blood sugar is chronically elevated and the body is not able to utilize glucose in its metabolism, it breaks down protein and fat for sustenance. For this reason I might add that, although I've gained weight, I haven't put on muscle mass at anywhere *near* the rate a normal person would."

Another diabetic found that diabetes interfered with his football because "I feel that I would have weighed much more had it not been for this disease. I guess I really weigh enough to play for a small college, but I had dreamed of being heavier and playing for Alabama. Still, I guess that I should be happy with what I have accomplished. I do get tired a little quicker than anyone else, but I try to never let it show. I'll never stop because of diabetes."

Even Joe Brink, who, as anyone can plainly see from his picture, has built up more muscle mass than most "normal" persons would ever dream of, thinks that diabetes is holding him back to some extent. "My diabetes, I feel, keeps me from getting the muscle size I really want. I can lose ten pounds in one day from exercising with weights and it's hard for me to maintain my weight. . . . Once you've won a title, as I have, you want to achieve the next step, which in my case would be Mr. Ohio. But I am not big enough or muscular enough to achieve this and I blame it on diabetes."

Dr. Olson, however, believes that even this muscle mass disadvantage is not necessarily necessary. He assures us that there is no reason that a diabetic can't put on muscle mass if he takes up weight training and similar muscle-building exercises, providing his diabetes is well controlled and his blood sugar is as close to normal as possible.

LOSE A FEW, WIN A FEW

It's true that Joe Brink feels his diabetes keeps him from achieving more wins in competition, *but*—and with this we now change our tune to the happier song of how diabetes can actually be an advantage, can actually make you better at your sport than you would be without it.

"*But*," as Joe explains, "diabetes does help me to be more determined at my sport. *Without this I would not be where I am today.*" So here's the paradox. Although diabetes may—we still have faith in Joe's ability to triumph—*may* keep him from winning the title of Mr. Ohio, if it hadn't been for diabetes he wouldn't have become a weight lifter in the first place and had the determination to win the title of Mr. Cincinnati.

Dick Bernstein, although not engaged in competitive weight lifting, also recognizes this advantage. "The diabetes has, indeed, helped me be better at my sport simply because you might say I participate in my sport to keep

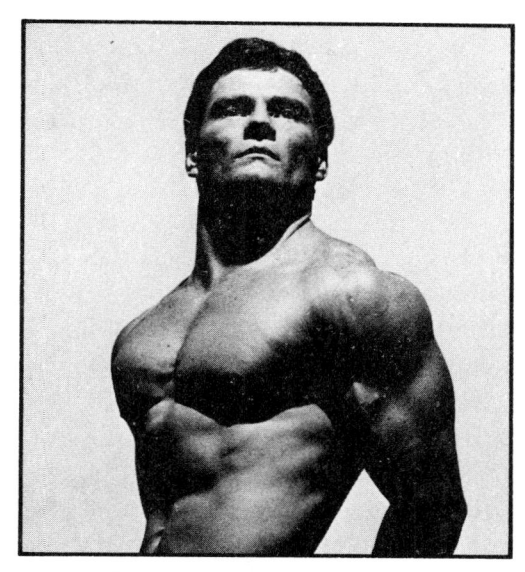

Joe Brink, flexing in his "Mr. Cincinnati" publicity photo, vividly shows that a diabetic can build up muscle mass. (Photo: Bob Lynn)

alive . . . at least to live longer, and there's enough incentive there to have made me very competent at it. In fact, I would say outstanding by comparison with other people that have worked out with me when I was in a public gymnasium."

When a person is, as Dick says and as Bill Talbert's book title put it, "playing for life," he does have a tendency to stick to it better.

The Backbone's Connected to the Pancreas. Many diabetics, though, don't consciously stick to their exercise just because they think it will make them live longer. The reason they stay with their walking or jogging or calisthenics —even when it's inconvenient or boring or they "just don't feel like it today"—is that they have developed the very valuable quality of self-discipline.

"I feel that diabetes has helped me in my sport because it has taught me self-discipline and made me adhere to a diet and exercise regime. I believe having a chronic disease tends to strengthen your backbone," says one.

This seems to be true. Hemophiliac Bobby Massie, the subject of his parents' book *Journey*, states, "When I conquer physical problems, I conquer many problems, and the defenses I have developed—like determination and patience—to deal with physical problems, I can apply to other problems as well."

Over and over diabetics have told us that the self-discipline they develop in diabetes carries over into other activities that require regularity and determination and stick-to-itiveness such as sports.

"I really think diabetes has helped in many ways and I think it has helped my family in the horse sport also, as we have accomplished much more since my diabetes; and I think it's because we have had to stabilize ourselves to some extent and become more serious and thereby conditioned our horses in the same way and made sure they were ready and able to compete in their classes. I think we took more time and had more discipline and made sure everything was fit and ready and took a more serious attitude toward competing than we would have otherwise."

"My skiing may have improved a little more than it might have otherwise, since I suspect that the fact that I have diabetes leads me to lose no opportunity to be out and at it."

"I'm a nineteen-year-old male diabetic who runs cross-country and track. I average a hundred miles of running per week all year round, except when I'm sick, of course. My best times in track are 4:39 for the one-mile run and 9:57 for the two-mile run. Both times are very competitive for my area, and very rarely do I finish out of the top two or three finishers in a race.

"The odd thing is that, since the discovery and control of my diabetes, my times have improved. My theory is that I can attribute this to more self-discipline and a better balanced diet."

This self-discipline carryover is not unique to chronic diseases, of course. Any time a person achieves self-discipline in one area of life, he can transfer it more easily to another. As an example, a friend of ours is related to a well-known harpsichordist. So involved was this musician with his music that he let himself go physically to the point that he could hardly waddle across the stage to his harpsichord at concerts. Then it happened that his doctor or his wife or he himself decided that it was ridiculous to be in this out-of-condition condition. He undertook a regular program of calisthenics and jogging. Gradually he worked himself up to a five-mile-a-day run plus the other exercises and he stuck to it—every day—just the way he stuck to practicing the harpsichord. He's now lean and lithe and feels great. Others who lacked his self-discipline might well have pooped out after the first week or so on the exercises. Olympic figure-skating champion Tenley Albright carried over her discipline on ice to medical school and is now a successful surgeon. So you see you don't have to be a diabetic to develop self-discipline, but diabetes *is* one way to get it.

The Healthiest Disease. On top of his self-discipline, an in-control diabetic has another ace in the sports-and-exercise deck: good health. "Ho, ho!" you may say. "What kind of garbage and other waste products are you giving me? A person with a disease, an incurable disease, has the advantage of good health?" Emphatically yes. Aside from her diabetes, June is about the healthiest person of her age we know. She just got an immaculate bill of health from her doctor on the occasion of her annual physical exam (blood pressure, 122/76; blood sugar, 88; cholesterol, 192; triglycerides, 76). The explanation for this is that she takes care of herself with excellent diet, regular hours, and —here we go again—exercise.

But you don't have to take our biased word for it. Take Mary Tyler Moore's: "I feel very positive about my 'malfunction.' It means I go to the doctor more than most people and exercise more than most people and watch my diet more than most people And as a consequence, I think I'm healthier than most people."

Or Thom Underwood's: "Man, this disease, this condition will keep you healthy and fit for whatever your heart desires. . . . I feel I'm better off because I'm not fat, never have I been out of shape, fitter at times than others and some of it is because I eat good and thoughtful."

Lots of other diabetics say the same thing:

"If you are a controlled diabetic and take care of yourself, you probably will discover that you are in far better health than your nondiabetic friends. By being on a controlled diet and regular exercise plus regular physicals, I find my health is excellent, any physical problems are picked up early, since regular checkups are necessary, and I find I am in much better physical shape than my friends."

"I always find myself running longer, swimming

faster, or playing tennis with more vigor and endurance. I can see why this is so because I don't eat any of the foods that so many people are faced with, e.g., cakes, cookies, snacks, and the many foods that are kept with artificial additives. Therefore the food I eat is put to good use and is capable of giving me the proper energy that I need during my sports."

"I do believe . . . that my diabetes has helped me in whatever sports I take up. I'm now getting on to middle years and I find that my weight hasn't climbed, primarily because my diet is excellent. Diabetes forces me to be in better shape."

"Diabetes, if you really think about it, makes a person become more aware of his body, especially what's good and bad for it. If you want to feel good, you eat good things. If you want to feel bad all the time, it's not hard."

Proof Positive. Another reason some diabetics may be better at their sport than they would be without their diabetes is that, when they participate in it, they're doing more than just playing a game and they're proving more than just their athletic prowess or endurance. Bill Talbert says, "I feel diabetes has helped me with my tennis. It has made me work a little harder to prove a point." Others agree:

"Diabetes makes me want to prove myself as good as or better than the guy next to me. It forces me to try harder."

"Maybe being a diabetic has made me work a little harder at what I do. I think a lot of people are still very uneducated about diabetes, and maybe because of this I felt I had to prove myself to them. I personally do not feel any different from anyone else, but because of beliefs people have about diabetes I may have had to put more of an effort toward things I do just to prove that I am no different."

"Yes, diabetes has helped me be better at my sport from a psychological point of view. I desire to compete and do better than the other old men! I am not ashamed of being a diabetic and do my best to convince young diabetics and parents of diabetic children that diabetes is not something to be feared and it need not lead to premature death."

"Maybe diabetes has not made me better at the sport itself, but it has made me more determined to be able to do things physically that were considered to be a no-no for a diabetic."

"It probably helps me in another sense. . . . There is always the feeling that you're representing a group of people—namely, diabetics who may be considered to be inferior—and there's a feeling here that you'll show the rest of the team or your competitors that you're not inferior and therefore you may try a little harder than the next guy to win or put in a good showing."

Naturally, not every diabetic is trying to prove anything with his sports and exercise. Free spirit and freethinker Thom Underwood has no hidden proof motives in his activities. "I don't have to prove myself to anyone," he says. "I enjoy what I do. I ski, climb, get out on a filthy, dusty trail, all of it's movement, speeds, or seeing country. The woods are my place for a little thinking and writing, playing a game or living a dream. I'm a mountain man for a couple of days. . . . I love to ski. . . . It's the speed, creative expression, fluidity of movement, rhythm. It is the sport that gives you the high, the satisfaction, the abnormal thing in life that keeps you healthy for the regular routines."

No Excuse for Diabetes. Then we come to a diabetes sports advantage that hardly anybody takes. This is using your diabetes as an excuse for flubbing up at a sport. "Gosh, that's a handy excuse," says Dave Engerbretson. " 'Well, I coulda beat you but my blood sugar was getting low.' I used to say this just as a standing joke. We'd play three games and that third game, if I got beat, that was the joke, but of course everybody *knew* it was a joke."

Most diabetics, though, won't even consider using diabetes as a for-real excuse. "My diabetes isn't responsible for anything," Ron Santo often stated during his years on the Cubs. "Just because I strike out doesn't mean I'm having an insulin reaction."

When we asked other diabetics if they had ever lost a sports competition because of diabetes, we got answers like:

"I lost a few first places in diving because of my own shortcomings and lack of skill, but never because of diabetes."

"I've lost plenty of sport competitions but never because of diabetes. Maybe a poor backhand but not because of diabetes."

"Saying you lost because of diabetes is an excuse for not playing up to your fullest capacity. If the diabetes is under control, coordination should not be affected. Again, I add adamantly, diabetes is not an excuse. Of course, if I miss a goal by a wide margin I can jokingly say my diabetes is affecting my eyesight today!"

"I have never lost due to my illness. If I ever should some day due to low blood sugar, I would blame it on myself for being stupid in planning and not on being diabetic."

Even when low blood sugar is a valid reason for losing, most diabetics still won't mention it to competitors.

"I expected to win a golf match, but at the final few holes I was looking at three balls and felt so desperate that I tried closing one eye. But the reaction caught up with me, and I lost the match. The opponent never knew I was a diabetic. She won 'fairly and squarely.'"

Double-Header. In participating in sports, some diabetics report that they find it a two-way field in which you can score a touchdown in both directions at the same time. Your sport makes you better at playing and winning the diabetes game, and your diabetes makes you a better sportsperson.

"I had to prove to myself that I could participate in a sport such as skiing or snowshoeing, and this gave me a lot of confidence in mastering my diabetes."

"I enjoy skiing and first-aid work a great deal. Trying to be neither arrogant nor modest, I am a good skier. I believe, when I began my patrol work four years ago, I became a more serious skier than ever before, realizing my diabetic way of life and knowing that in order to enjoy and be successful at my patrol work I would have to be in full control of my diabetes. I believe one hand has washed the other. I am in full control of myself on the mountain and am good at what I do."

Pro-spective. For people who are really involved with sports, involved to the extent that they are highly skilled at the sport and perhaps have the goal of going pro, diabetes can be advantageous in keeping sports in perspective. When you're a champion athlete, there's the possibility that you can start regarding "the toy department of life" as the whole department store.

A diabetic whose disease was discovered when she was a star tennis player at Brigham Young University explains, "Diabetes made me realize that tennis isn't the whole world, and maybe my value system was getting a little unbalanced. Tennis, competing, traveling, and all the attention and publicity we would get was beginning to affect me in such a way that it was all I lived for."

FINAL SCORE

So, OK, when you total out the pluses and minuses, what's the score? Does diabetes hinder or help a person as far as sports are concerned? The answer to that question is up to you. It all boils down to the way you play the game. It's as one fifteen-year-old female hockey player says: "You have to have it in your heart, not in your insulin."

Appendixes

Appendix A

Diabetic Doers' Profiles

These are some of the people who shared their experiences in sports and diabetes with us during the spring of 1975 and whose words and deeds appear on the pages of this book. We think you will agree that, whether or not they have the trophies and ribbons to prove it, every one is a winner.

CLARA ADAMS, Sun City, California. Age 79. Diabetic for 4 years. Treatment: diet and pills. Sport: lawn bowling. "My exercise keeps me from gaining weight and my diabetes makes my bowling better because I am more careful of my diet."

THOMAS JOSEPH ALARIE, West Warwick, Rhode Island. Age 13. Diabetic for 3 years. Treatment: 45–50 units of NPH insulin. Sports: baseball, football, basketball. "When I scored three touchdowns in one game in football and I scored the most points in one of my basketball games, I felt I have taken complete and total control of my diabetes and it has not taken control over me."

JUNE ALBERT, Wolcott, Connecticut. Age 24. Diabetic for 1 year. Treatment: Orinase and D.B.I. Sports: tennis, bike riding, swimming, gym, jogging, ice skating, skiing. "Being a diabetic will give you opportunities and insights into learning things you wouldn't have been exposed to otherwise. Life will have a different meaning to you. Being diabetic opens a whole new thinking in you. You'll probably wonder now, What am I capable of doing or not doing? What is my potential? I'm very certain if I were not a diabetic I would know myself much less well than I do now."

TIM W. ANDERSON, Bellingham, Washington. Age 20. Diabetic for 4 years. Treatment: NPH insulin. Sports: skiing (cross-country and downhill), tennis, volleyball, baseball, mountain climbing, water sports, all camping activities, backpacking, jogging. "You need no favors or special help. Prove yourself as you are—just as good as or better than the next guy. Use diabetes as a positive direction toward a healthy disciplined body, not as a crutch."

BETSY AUSTIN, Lincoln, Massachusetts. Age 17. Diabetic for 8 years. Treatment: insulin. Sports: skiing (cross-country and downhill), tennis, swimming, field hockey, sailing. "A person who regards diabetes as a handicap, or something that must be overcome, does not understand diabetes and has not accepted it as part of his/her life. It is a part and should become something as accepted as your knees!"

CHRIS BANKS, Burnaby, British Columbia. Age 25. Diabetic for 10 years. Treatment: insulin. Sports: skiing, jogging, badminton, football. "Never use diabetes as an excuse for not making it to the heights to which you have aspired."

VIRGINIA MAGGIO BEAMSDERFER, Gorham, New York. Age 24. Diabetic for 16 years. Treatment: insulin. Sports: field hockey, tennis, swimming, archery, bowling, all sports required for P.E. degree; currently a physical education teacher. "Don't let diabetes complicate your life. Being diabetic does not mean you are any less skilled or capable of participating in a sport. The choice is yours: live a normal life or live one in which you feel you need added protection."

RICHARD K. BERNSTEIN, Mamaroneck, New York. Age 41. Diabetic for 30 years. Treatment: insulin. Sports: weight lifting, body building, boating, sailing, rowing, jogging. "If I had two messages to give to diabetics, at least to juvenile-onset diabetics, I would encourage daily strenuous sports activity and I would encourage multiple daily blood-sugar determinations."

PAUL T. BISESTI, Longmeadow, Massachusetts. Age 35. Diabetic for 12 years. Treatment: insulin. Sports: running, downhill skiing, hiking, weight lifting. "Diabetics need more exposure—as most Americans do—to the need for greater physical fitness."

JANET BLACK, Pocatello, Idaho. Age 40. Diabetic for 10 years. Treatment: 40 units NPH insulin. Sports: skiing, tennis. "All diabetic sportspeople know the importance of sugar. The thing I learned the hard way is don't just have it *in* you—have it *on* you as well."

MARK A. BLACKBURN, Indianapolis, Indiana. Age 22. Diabetic for 2 years. Treatment: insulin. Sports: basketball, camping, hiking, skiing. "Diabetes is an inconvenience, not a disease to worry about all the time. In a way a person with diabetes should be thankful he isn't hooked up to a kidney dialysis machine or doesn't have a disorder that would keep him or her away from any sport or work."

JOE BRINK, Cincinnati, Ohio. Age 30. Diabetic for 20 years. Treatment: insulin. Sports: baseball and football in high school, weight lifting. "I feel very strongly that *any* diabetic can do anything he wants to do with the proper instruction and encouragement. I think most diabetics think they are invalids and this is so ridiculous. Diabetics need to be told and convinced that they *can* lead normal lives if they take care of themselves. A change in mental attitude, I believe, would make a world of difference in their lives."

JOAN LINN BRUTSCHE, Greenville, Ohio. Age 40. Diabetic for 12 years. Treatment: insulin. Sports: jumping rope, biking, swimming, tennis, canoeing. "I'm sure diabetes hasn't been a handicap for me in the area of physical activity because I have continued to keep up physically and am able to do most active things without muscle soreness or fatigue as other nondiabetics experience."

LAILA M. CAMPBELL, Manning Park, British Columbia. Age 29. Diabetic for 7 years. Treatment: 50 units NPH insulin. Sports: skiing, hiking, biking, swimming, tennis. "The main thing is don't be afraid to try—nothing is impossible until you prove it impossible. The second thing, and what I still struggle with, is to be able to accept your limits; but remember that other people have limits, too, and other people get tired, too. It's not just because you're diabetic."

DAVE CAREY, Lake Forest, Illinois. Age 27. Diabetic for 17 years. Treatment: 42 units Lente insulin. Sport: skiing.

"I don't consider diabetes a handicap. It has nothing to do with the thrill I get from skiing. Diabetes is just 'me,' while skiing is something that I work at and love."

JOHN E. CASS, Van Nuys, California. Age 50. Diabetic for 11 years. Treatment: insulin, oral medication (D.B.I.). Sports: long-distance running, golf, skin and scuba diving. "We have a chronic disease that requires us to have medication, diet, sleep, and exercise to exist. With the knowledge of this we have a 'built-in discipline.' If we let this 'built-in discipline' work for us, we can lower our dosage of medication and have a sense of well-being and confidence that no one can take away from us."

BRENT CLARK, Nampa, Idaho. Age 18. Diabetic for 5 years. Treatment: insulin. Sports: cross-country running, basketball, track. "If you want to do something but diabetes scares you off, you don't want to do it bad enough. There is always a way to do it, if you just try. It may take something to get used to it, there may be some problems to work out, but *it can be done!*"

GAIL DIETZ CONLEY, Trenton, New Jersey. Age 23. Diabetic for 17 years. Treatment: Lente insulin. Sport: bicycling. "As long as I know my limits, I feel that I can do anything I want to try. I know a diabetic who bicycled 900 miles from Illinois to New Jersey in ten days. . . . If you're having trouble with reactions or are afraid of having problems, don't be afraid to ask other people for help and reassurance. Do not let yourself feel bullied into straining yourself more than you can handle."

JERRY M. COOPER, Helena, Montana. Age 23. Diabetic for 10 years. Treatment: 50 units NPH insulin. Sports:

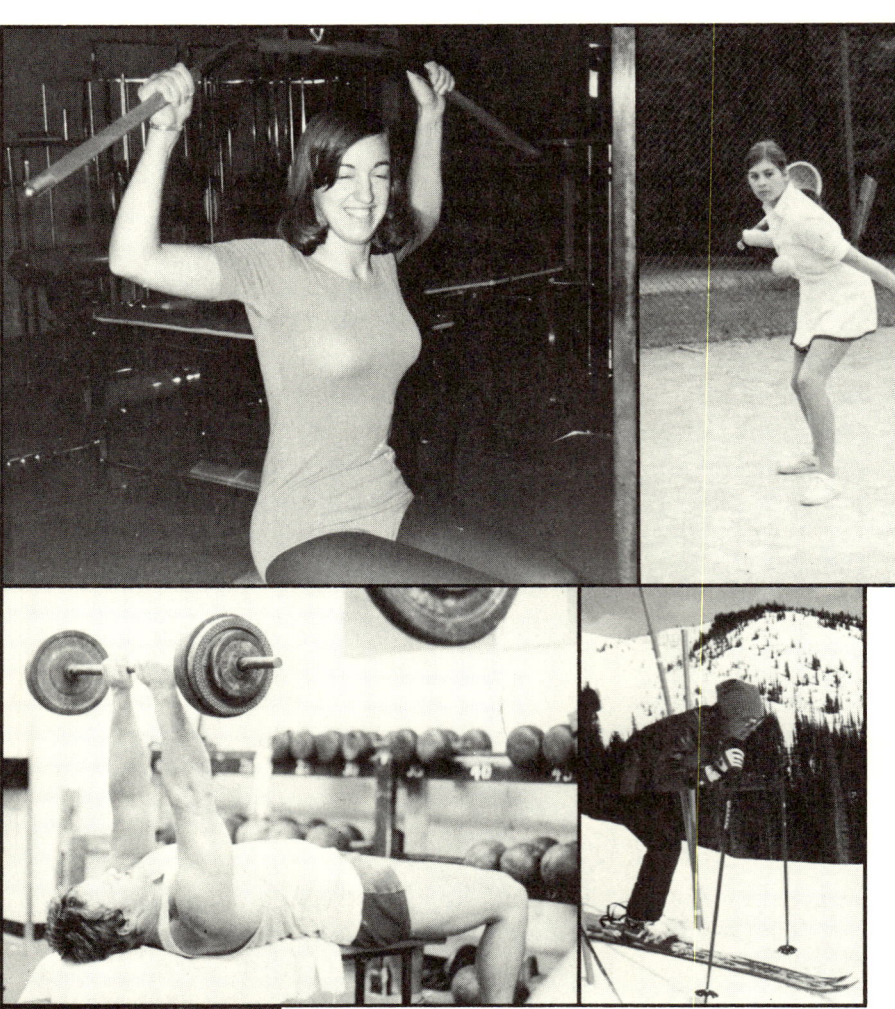

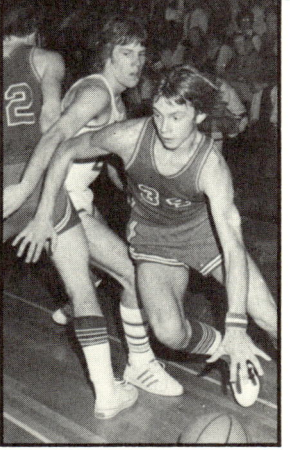

From left to right, top to bottom: June Albert, Betsy Austin, Joe Brink, Laila Campbell, and Brent Clark.

skiing, swimming, backpacking, hiking. "I do not feel I have a handicap. That is something in your head. . . . Participating in sports is probably the best thing you can do for yourself."

NORMA CREIGHTON, San Jose, California. Age 58. Diabetic for 10 years. Treatment: insulin. Sports: skiing and golf. "Don't sit back and let life pass you by. Work out the problems of diabetes with the doctor, lead as normal a life as possible, and participate. And don't feel sorry for yourself—there is always someone with more serious problems."

ROBERT KEITH CROWLING, Norfolk, Virginia. Age 23. Diabetic for 21½ years. Treatment: insulin. Sports: karate (blue belt), skiing, sailing, football, baseball, basketball, tennis, surfing, handball, motorcycling, backpacking. "You will never find out just what you are capable of if you take the attitude of 'It is better to have never tried and never failed than to have tried and failed.' . . . My diabetes does not cause me fear when I am active. I am cautious, but that comes naturally due to just knowing that I am a diabetic. Diabetes is a way of life to me. I have learned to use my senses in ways that people without this condition would not have to."

GREGORY CUTTER, San Diego, California. Age 20. Diabetic for 5 years. Treatment: insulin. Sports: skiing, hiking, sailing, flying (power and glider), scuba diving, body surfing, motorcycling. "Diabetes is *not a handicap*. It is just biochemistry and most of all a state of mind which can be good or bad. With a good state of mind nothing can stop you. With a bad state of mind you're never going to be anything else but a diabetic."

ANNA DEVINE, Phillipsburg, New Jersey. Age 68. Diabetic for 1 year and 4 months. Treatment: diet. Sport: archery. "No problems in my sport. I'm OK. I feel good all the time. Everything is my pleasure. I have won about 150 awards in my sport."

RICHARD CHARLES DRISCOLL, Hazlet, New Jersey. Age 19. Diabetic for 2 years. Treatment: 30 units of NPH insulin. "Diabetes is not that bad and you can beat it. It doesn't take much: love of life, love of people, pride in oneself and one's own ability, determination to conquer a disease. Just put your mind and body toward your goal in life and do it! I have found hope in this Bible quotation: 'If thou canst believe, all things are possible to him that believeth' (Mark 9:23)."

DAVID L. ENGERBRETSON, Moscow, Idaho. Age 39. Diabetic for 16 years. Treatment: insulin. Sports: skiing (cross-country and downhill), backpacking, canoeing, camping, fly fishing, jogging, spelunking, sailplaning, sportscar rallye driving, bowling, hunting. "The diagnosis of diabetes is not a condemnation. But the diabetic who does not learn all he can about the disease, and his own response to it, is in for a bad time of it both physically and mentally. With an understanding of it, and with cautious experimentation, the diabetic can lead the kind of life he wants to."

DICK EPLEY, South Ogden, Utah. Age 28. Diabetic for 20 years. Treatment: insulin. Sports: skiing, golfing, hunting, fishing. "A diabetic should not be ashamed of his condition or resentful. Each day should be lived and thought of as a gift. Let your friends know you are a diabetic and how they can help you. Hasn't everyone had a friend they have helped out, or wished they had known something about a friend so they could help out?"

ELAINE ESTES, San Jose, California. Age 16. Diabetic for 2 years. Treatment: Insulin. Sports: track, tennis, water skiing, skiing, all seasonal sports. "I refuse to let myself fall under the category of being handicapped. If you as a diabetic put yourself in this category you will get into a rut. You will become inactive and fat. For me diabetes is only a reason to get involved with sports, stay on a balanced diet, and be healthy."

DOROTHY FRANK, Palm Desert, California. Age 64. Diabetic for 45 years. Treatment: insulin. Sports: walking, golf. "If you're interested in golf, diabetes should prove no obstacle. I think a participation in any active sport (or sports) is salutary for diabetic control and general good health."

LEE GERNER, Novato, California. Age 61. Diabetic for 20 years. Treatment: Orinase and D.B.I.; recently changed to a small amount of insulin. Sports: jogging, weight lifting, isometrics, and bicycling. "I have never felt any ill effects from my diabetes, and the doctors tell me it is because I am so active. My combined sports activity takes about two hours a day. Many days I do this in addition to eight hours of heavy physical labor. I weigh exactly the same and have the same measurements as when I was seventeen years old. I would like to say to all diabetics who do not have serious side effects to *exercise, exercise, exercise!*"

LISA GODFREY, Richmond, British Columbia. Age 11. Diabetic for 1½ years. Treatment: insulin. Sports: skiing, ice-skating, rollerskating, running, swimming, horseback riding. "Diabetics can take part in all sports without fear as long as diet and insulin requirements are adequate and regular habits are kept to as far as possible."

MARCIA GOODHART, Fresh Meadows, New York. Age 18. Diabetic for 14 years. Treatment: 52 units insulin. Sports: field hockey, softball, basketball, volleyball, badminton. "I have proved to myself that diabetes can be controlled and won't be an obstacle if it is watched. My message to other diabetics is not to let diabetes stop you from participating in *any* sports, including strenuous ones."

ROLF A. GOOS, South Lake Tahoe, California. Age 31. Diabetic for 20 years. Treatment NPH insulin. Sports: tennis, skiing, running. "Since taking up sports I feel a lot better. I know that my body needs it. If I don't exercise for a few days, I feel tired and weary very easily. The minute I go out in the fresh air and do my exercise it's like a booster. I look better, I feel better, and the food tastes better."

JOHN GORNELL, Allendale, New Jersey. Age 34. Diabetic for 5 years. Treatment: 30 units NPH insulin. Sports: tennis, skiing, platform tennis (in 1974 was ranked, with partner, sixteenth in the nation). "Don't let diabetes prevent your active participation in sports. Participate without any feeling of being inferior."

SANDRA FAY HAGE, Hanska, Minnesota. Age 18. Diabetic for 11 years. Treatment: insulin. Sports: track, basketball, swimming, volleyball, softball, skating, skiing, tobogganing, bicycling, hiking, camping. "Set your goals and work toward them, because you can do it if you really try. You

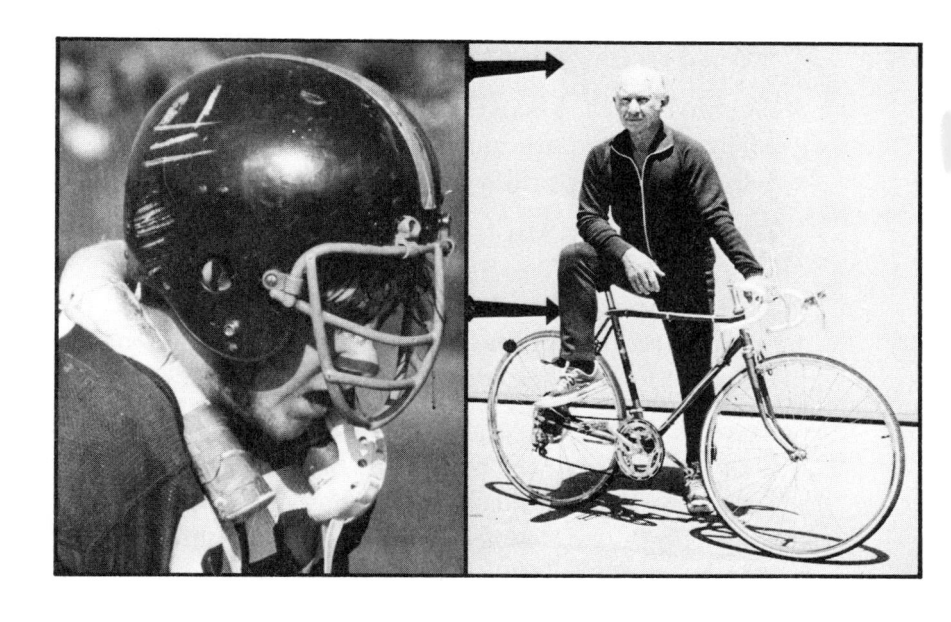

Above, Rich Driscoll, Lee Gerner; below, Marcia Goodhart, Rolf Goos.

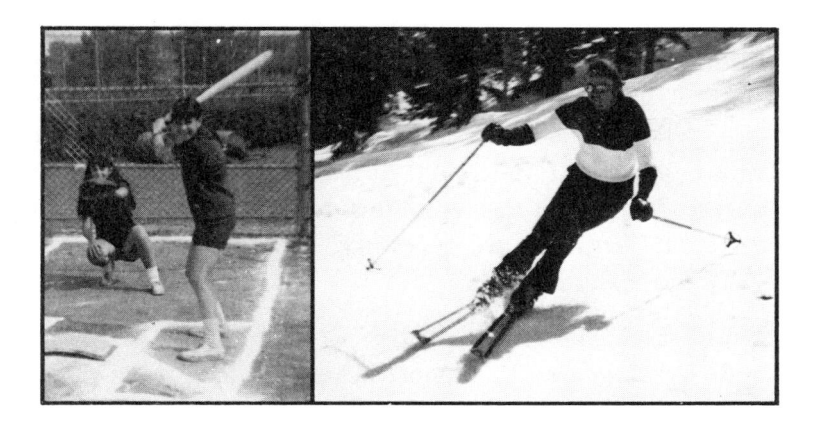

shouldn't worry about anything because you'll learn to adapt and there are many others around you willing to help. Best wishes to all you sports-oriented diabetics."

THERESA HARRIS, Mission Viejo, California. Age 17. Diabetic for 1 year. Treatment, insulin. Sports: waterskiing, motorcycling, scuba diving. "After I found out I had diabetes, I actually became more active than ever. I really do love my life and I wouldn't trade it for anyone else's."

VINCE E. HAVLICAK, American Falls, Idaho. Age 16. Diabetic for 11 years. Treatment: 54 units NPH insulin. Sports: Weight lifting, rodeo riding, basketball, skiing, waterskiing, swimming, hunting, motorcycling. "There are always people worse off than you've ever thought of being. Some people have a bigger handicap and aren't sick physically, if you know what I mean. Diabetes is not so bad; besides, it's about all I've ever known. I can do whatever I want to try. Pretty darn good life, I'd say."

KAREN HAYES, Hudson, Massachusetts. Age, in 20s. Diabetic for 4 years. Treatment: insulin. Sports: skiing, cycling, swimming. "Diet and exercise is the most effective method of controlling a diabetic, even if you are on insulin. I feel better and have a much easier time staying controlled while on a regular program of sports and exercise. When I don't have time to devote to this, my sugar runs higher and I notice that I don't seem to have as much energy. When getting a great deal of exercise, even though certain adjustments are necessary, I feel far better physically and mentally."

ERIC HEAD, Mackenzie, British Columbia. Age 11. Diabetic for 1¾ years. Treatment: insulin. Sports: skiing, fishing, bike riding, tobogganing, floor hockey. "The main thing is to be as normal as all the other kids."

MIKE HICKS, Flagstaff, Arizona. Age 15. Diabetic for 7 months. Treatment: insulin. Sports: football, baseball, wrestling. "Having diabetes made me try harder to prove I can still do it. Be careful and don't get discouraged. As long as you're careful you can do anything anyone else can."

ERIC WADE HILTS, De Witt, Michigan. Age 14. Diabetic for 10½ years. Treatment 26 units Lente insulin. Sports: wrestling, golf, baseball, swimming, canoeing, kayaking, chess. "The sport that gives me the most satisfaction is wrestling, for when I come off the mat and have won another match, I know I am the strongest and best trained of the two boys out there. I do not feel that diabetes is a handicap in a sports event."

JACQUELINE HOPKINS, Chula Vista, California. Age 19. Diabetic for 4 years. Treatment: insulin. Sports: skiing, golf, tennis. "A person must not be led to feel like a freak or a china doll. If a diabetic gets involved in sports he can feel like a normal person and better cope with his disease. The more active a diabetic is the better his overall health will be."

DICK HUMPHREYS, Kirkwood, Pennsylvania. Age 32. Diabetic for 18 years. Treatment: insulin. Sports: tennis, Ping-Pong, backpacking, jogging, bicycling. "The late Abraham Maslow writes of how we should compare what we can do with the outstanding members of our race, not the average. Try to achieve on a level with the best—the fastest runner, the saint, the most creative artist. Then, even if we do fall short, it's still much better than just average."

RICHARD JOHNSON, Webster, New York. Age 32. Diabetic for 23 years. Treatment: insulin. Sports: golf, skiing. "Diabetes is a nuisance but certainly not a severe handicap. Sports were made for diabetics!"

BETSY KADWIT, Milwaukee, Wisconsin. Age 13½. Diabetic for 4 years. Treatment: insulin. Sports: basketball, tennis, waterskiing, snow skiing, track. "Don't let diabetes keep you from doing anything. There is always a way to work things out. If you can't find a way to work it out, then consult your doctor or your local diabetes association. It is always worth the extra effort. Every diabetic should certainly be very active and not hesitate to participate in all sports. Just don't brush your diabetes away during activity; take care of it and handle it."

ALAN S. KALKIN, Canoga Park, California. Age 41. Diabetic 7 years. Treatment: insulin. Sports: karate, four-wall handball, running, weight training. "Have a good spirit. By this I mean: enjoy life! Although diabetes is a definite factor, it is but one facet. With good spirit and determination life can be full, thereby reducing the impact of diabetes on your life."

JOYCE V. KRUEGER, Rib Lake, Wisconsin. Age 36. Diabetic for 12 years. Treatment: insulin. Sports: showing horses, training horses (high-schooled trick horses and show horses), teaching horsemanship to 4-H members; certified state horse show judge. "Get out and try no matter how you feel at the moment. Put out the effort. Nothing is gained without effort. It's like me or anyone getting up at

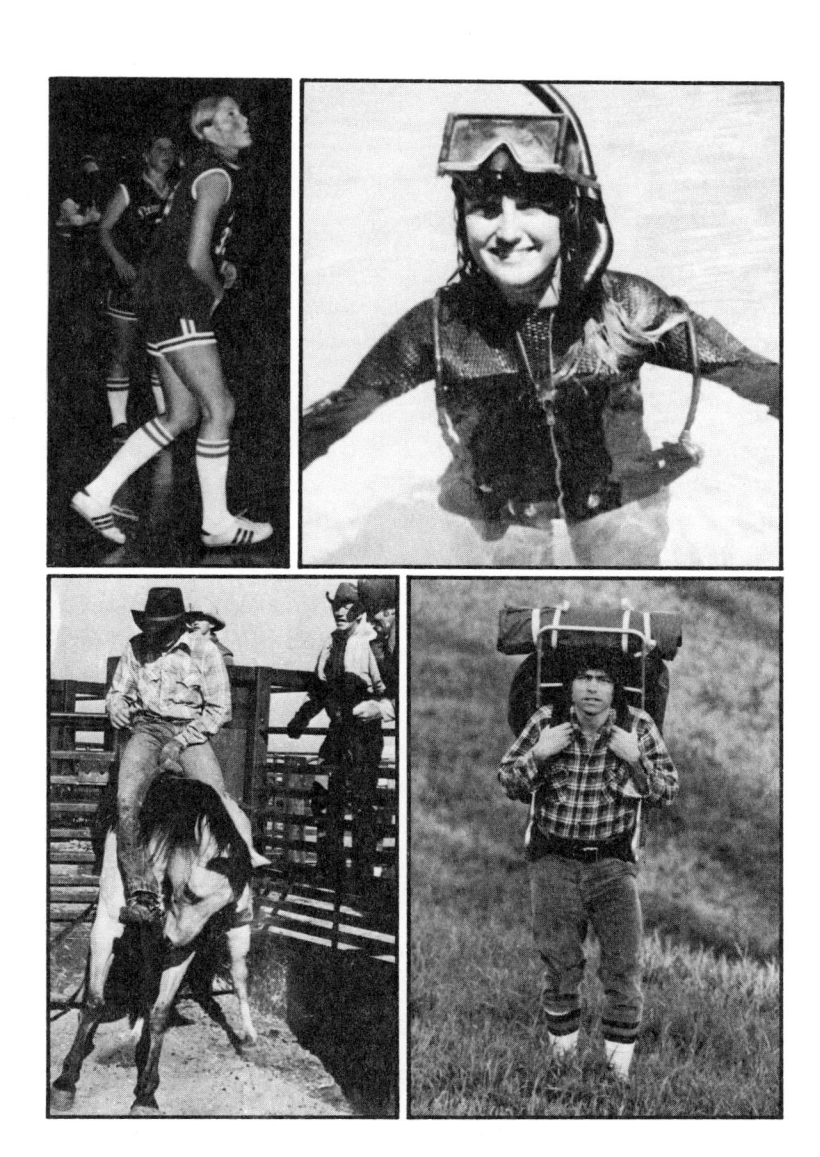

*Above, Sandra Fay Hage, Theresa Harris;
below, Vince Havlicak, Dick Humphreys.*

3 A.M. to get ready for a horse show. You would much rather stay in bed, but once you are at the show, you are so glad that you made the effort."

MARNIE LAWLOR, Waterbury, Connecticut. Age 19. Diabetic for 7 years. Treatment: 40 units insulin. Sports: tennis, swimming, running. "If it weren't for diabetes I know I wouldn't have the interest in sports that I do. I never get down on myself because I have diabetes. I have diabetes and I accept that. I also accept the fact that I am a lot better off than some people who don't. . . . If sports are in the picture, don't hesitate to get into that picture."

EDWARD LEETE, Minneapolis, Minnesota. Age 46. Diabetic for 17 years. Treatment: 50 units Lente insulin. Sports: long-distance running, skiing (cross-country and downhill). "It is often said that diabetics age more rapidly than nondiabetics. I believe that this process can be reversed by long-distance running. I believe that many of the characteristics of old age can be postponed indefinitely by energetic exercise."

MURIEL LINDERHOLM, Edina, Minnesota. Age 48. Diabetic for 17 years. Treatment: 17 units semi-Lente insulin. Sports: tennis, walking, skiing (cross-country and downhill). "Exercise is the most important thing that a diabetic can do to improve his or her well-being. It keeps everything circulating in your body, keeps your muscles in tone, utilizes glucose in muscle cells, and gives one a healthy mental attitude. I have seen diabetics who treat themselves as invalids and this is so wrong. I can do anything I want to do and am able to keep up with any of my nondiabetic friends in all activities."

Diabetic Doers' Profiles 221

SHELLY LOWENKOPF, Santa Barbara, California. Age 44. Diabetic for 5 years. Treatment: diet and exercise. Sports: hiking, running. "Of course the diabetic is 'different.' If he or she follows a sensible regime of diet and exercise, he or she will live longer and feel better than most civilians. ... Diabetes is a blessing in disguise and sports is a perfect way to discover the blessing."

STEPHEN JON LURIE, New York, New York. Age 18. Diabetic for 8 years. Treatment: insulin. Sports: tennis, golf, skiing. "With proper training and awareness of your own limits and capabilities, there is nothing a diabetic can't do. Exercise is very important in a diabetic's life. If a diabetic wants to play a sport, he or she should be given all the chances in the world to play it to the fullest."

THOMAS M. MCGURRIN, Beverly Hills, California. Age 46. Diabetic for 8 years. Treatment: insulin. Sports: skiing, backpacking, horseback riding, fishing, swimming. "My skiing ability has improved tremendously since I became a diabetic, and the fact that I can keep up with my children and others who are not diabetic gives me a great deal of satisfaction. I feel sports have helped me overcome some of the mental unhappiness that I originally experienced when I learned I had diabetes. Any diabetic who uses diabetes as an excuse not to engage in athletics is doing himself a disservice."

MIKE MCNALLY, Mechanicsburg, Pennsylvania. Age 28. Diabetic for 11 years. Treatment: 50 units NPH insulin. Sports: bicycling, running, tennis. "My control is lousy without exercise. Exercise is the key to my diabetic control. Participation in sports gives one a sense of normal living which is also healthy for the mind. I'd like to see group participation in sports activities for diabetics on an organized basis. Learning in a safe environment might encourage more diabetics to the athletic life."

MIKE MCNUTT, Birmingham, Michigan. Age 13. Diabetic for 3 years. Treatment: 20 units NPH insulin. Sports: tennis, skiing, sailing, basketball, baseball. "Always take time out to think about how you feel so you don't have a reaction. Diabetics can do any sport as any other person does. They are as capable."

TOM MARKOVICH, JR., Huntington, Pennsylvania. Age 25. Diabetic for 6 years. Treatment: 40 units NPH insulin. Sports: tennis, skiing, golf, basketball, swimming. "When I first became a diabetic I lived to enjoy sports, and I thought because I was a diabetic I would have to give up everything. I felt sorry for myself the first two or three weeks and moped around the house. But I finally told myself to try and see if it did make a difference. When I found out it didn't, I had it licked. Although being diabetic isn't the greatest thing in the world, it sure as hell isn't even close to being the worst."

MIKE MARTIN, Vancouver, British Columbia. Age 48. Diabetic for 5 years. Treatment: Insulin. Sports: skiing, hiking, camping, fishing, snowshoeing, golf. "I had to prove to myself that I could participate in a sport such as skiing or snowshoeing, and this gave me a lot of confidence in mastering my diabetes. A diabetic person can participate in many sports, either in competitive or recreational fields, once he has learned to live with his problem. And feeling sorry for himself or herself will only shorten the lifespan when you can be out enjoying life as any other person. Don't be a spectator. Get out and off your butts and enjoy life and participate in a sport of your choice even if it is only walking."

GLENN A. MATSON, Littleton, Colorado. Age 52. Diabetic for 20 years. Treatment: insulin. Sports: bicycle riding, skiing, hunting. "If diabetes is a handicap, I guess I just haven't heard about it. Maybe diabetes has offered an additional challenge to me to prove to myself that diabetes is not a deterrent or restriction. It may require some special planning and special requirements. With these satisfied, do your thing, whatever it may be."

JOHN MAXWELL, Spokane, Washington. Age 52. Diabetic for 5 years. Treatment: pills. Sports: walking, hiking, water-skiing, snow skiing. "I have become very sold on a regular sports program of physical activity and outdoor exercise. I am sure diabetes has had a strong influence on the development of a sports program simply because I have found I generally feel better. I am sure a regular routine of physical activity achieves that state rather than sporadic effort."

CAROL MENSES, El Paso, Texas. Age 38. Diabetic for 10 years. Treatment: insulin. Sports: skiing, swimming, golf. "I feel best when I am exercising. Inactivity makes me feel tired and listless whether my blood sugar is high or low. I can't think of anything worse than being inactive."

PATRICIA MOLL, Westminster, Colorado. Age 25. Diabetic for 9 years. Treatment: insulin. Sports: softball, field hockey, jogging, diving, skiing. "Participating in a sport and doing well in it has given me confidence in myself.

My experience in each sport has given me a better knowledge of my individual case of diabetes and how to keep it under control. Being active in sports has given me confidence in being able to adjust my diet and insulin dosage accordingly. Exercising also makes me feel so much better physically. It brightens my outlook! By participating in each of my sports I feel that I have more or less conquered my disease. I don't look at diabetes as a handicap. It is more like a minor inconvenience."

BRIAN MORRIS, Bramlea, Ontario. Age 9½. Diabetic for 4 years. Treatment: insulin. Sports: baseball, bowling, skiing, ice skating. "I feel that sports and eventually competition in sports help control my diabetes. Keep active!"

STEPHEN NARUK, Middletown, Connecticut. Age 20. Diabetic for 11 years. Treatment: insulin. Sports: swimming, bicycling, sailing, rock climbing, skiing (cross-country and downhill), tennis. "I don't think that I've ever considered my diabetes in particular as a handicap. Becoming a diabetic at age eight or nine and having to face the prospect of being on a diet and taking 'needles' for the rest of one's life is, at that age, very hard to accept; but in retrospect it's perhaps better to become diabetic at that age than any other because one adapts to it so quickly then—nobody is prone to brooding over one's fate at that age, as one might at twenty, I think—and one can't look back and sulk about what might have been if one was not diabetic. . . . Don't let it stop you from doing anything, ever."

BRIAN ANTHONY NELSON, New York, New York. Age 17. Diabetic for 2 years. Treatment: insulin. Sports: rugby, fencing, swimming, skiing. "You should never hold back in fear of your diabetes, but you also should never ignore it either."

CYNTHIA NOTTINGHAM, Franktown, Virginia. Age 18. Diabetic for 8 years. Treatment: insulin. Sports: riding horses, softball, volleyball, basketball, football. "Never give up because sports are for everybody. Being a diabetic makes you a special person. Being a diabetic athlete makes you even more special. It shows people you had enough strength and courage to face your problem and overcome it."

PATRICIA OSGOOD, Kearsarge, New Hampshire. Age 47. Diabetic for 7 years. Treatment: insulin. Sports: cross-country skiing, hiking, mountain climbing, jogging, canoeing, bowling. "The fearful work of getting and staying in good physical condition is worth all the effort it may take. . . . When I first learned that I was diabetic I was completely dominated by the fact. This state of mind soon became discouraging, not to say depressing. A number of factors contributed to the gradual lessening of the stronghold which diabetes had upon me, but I think that finding that I could still pursue the sports I most enjoyed just as vigorously as before perhaps did more than anything to restore my drooping spirits."

SUSAN PINE, Gibbstown, New Jersey. Age 13. Diabetic for 11 years. Treatment: insulin. Sports: running, swimming, track events, skiing. "I do not consider diabetes a handicap. You are just like everyone else except you have to watch yourself. . . . I think all diabetics should join up in teams or sports things."

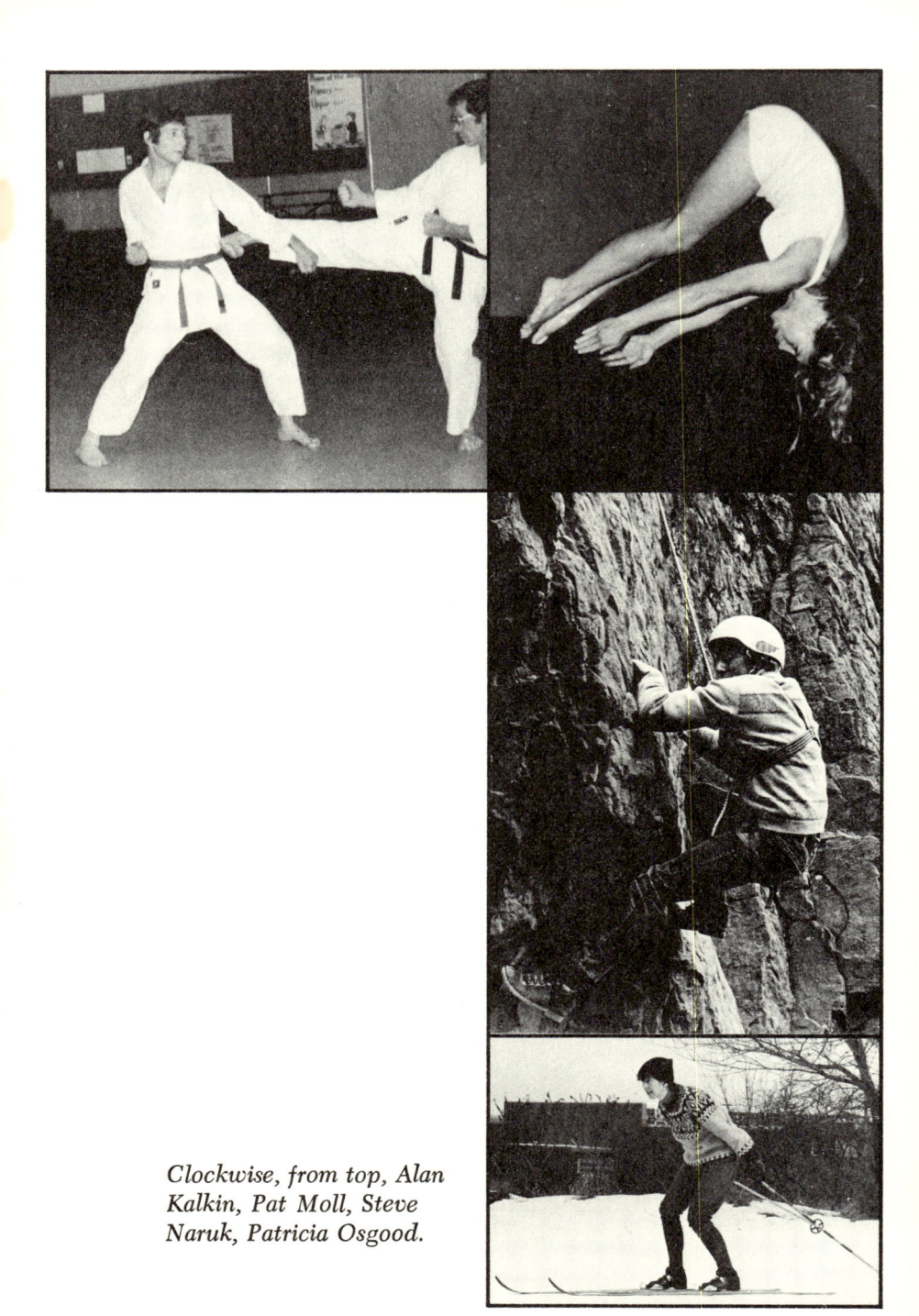

Clockwise, from top, Alan Kalkin, Pat Moll, Steve Naruk, Patricia Osgood.

HELEN PIRMAN, Alexandria, Kentucky. Age 67. Diabetic for 10 years. Treatment: pills. Sports: kite flying, walking, fishing. "At first one is frightened and feels life must be lived very differently, but such is not the case. . . . Do the things you are supposed to do, and go ahead with life as others do. Some are worse off than you. Don't feel sorry for yourself or expect special favors on account of whatever ails you."

BECKI QUINN, San Bernardino, California. Age 20. Diabetic for 9 years. Treatment: insulin. Sports: karate, water-skiing, snow skiing, miscellaneous exercises. "I have never not done something because I am a diabetic. I never worry about hurting myself because if I did I probably wouldn't do anything."

KENNETH R. REEDER, Wilmington, Delaware. Age 34. Diabetic for 15 years. Treatment: insulin. Sports: volleyball, basketball, golf. "Each time I don a pair of sneakers I feel I have conquered diabetes. I feel that the rigorous way in which I have participated in sports has been greatly beneficial to me. When I begin to feel poorly as a result of spilling sugar I get to exercising in order to feel better."

BOB RIEGER, Toronto, Ontario. Age 31. Diabetic for 17 years. Treatment: insulin. Sports: horseback riding, skiing, show jumping, horse training, squash, badminton. "A person with diabetes can't really allow it to stop him from doing the things he wants to do. You've just got to learn to live with it and it should not really hold you back from doing any kind of sports activity that you want to do."

FRANK H. ROBLES, Salt Lake City, Utah. Age 45. Diabetic

for 15 years. Treatment: insulin. Sports: skiing, backpacking, jogging, tennis, golf. "None of us lives in a vacuum and those who are not interested in taking care of themselves because, as they state, 'I'm only hurting myself,' must realize that others who develop diabetes very often are influenced by people whom they know have had diabetes for some time. If we are poorly controlled and have great difficulties . . . we give other people including other diabetics the feeling that it is a terrific handicap. I've talked to many diabetics who have been very badly influenced by another diabetic's example. We do influence other people and since we do we should try to make that influence beneficial."

Jo ROSENBERG, Laguna Hills, California. Age 64. Diabetic for 29 years. Treatment: insulin. Sports: swimming, walking, biking. "My diabetes has made me healthier because it makes me eat better and take better care of myself."

DURWOOD B. ROWLEY, Millis, Massachusetts. Age 46. Diabetic for 22 years. Treatment: insulin. Sports: tennis, bowling, hiking, gardening. "I have always been interested and participated in sports. My continued active participation is probably due somewhat to my being a diabetic and the value of exercise in maintaining good control. You will also meet many fine people and establish good friends by participating in sports."

R. J. RYAN, Long Beach, California. Age 42. Diabetic for 13 years. Treatment: insulin. Sports: bicycling, handball, jogging, hiking, camping, motorcycling. "Being able to cycle 100 miles in a little over six hours makes me feel pretty good. I've taken groups out on hikes and after several miles wound up carrying some of the younger ones, and some of the packs of adults that gave out, yet enjoy all around better health than I do. . . . It seems that diabetics are prone to certain problems, heart trouble, poor circulation, etc. The heart is a muscle. Exercise just keeps it in shape."

DEBORAH LYNN SCHLAPPAL, Willowick, Ohio. Age 22. Diabetic for 12 years. Treatment: insulin. Sports: bowling, skiing, bicycling. "There is no difference between me and the girl putting her skis on next to me. There is no difference between me and the woman bowling on the next alley. There is no difference between me and the girl riding that bike. Diabetics do have their own group, but I'd say that's the foundation of our basic life. After we talked and learned from others in our same group, then it's time to go out and conquer the world."

DEAN SCHMETTER, Hobart, Indiana. Age 17. Diabetic for 1 year. Treatment: insulin. Sports: golf, hunting, fishing, hiking. "Put out the idea that diabetes will hinder you. You can do anything even with your problem. Don't ever use it as an excuse. Don't feel life is over. Show people that you can succeed."

ARLENE MARGARET SCHOLER, New Hyde Park, New York. Age 34. Diabetic for 11 years. Treatment: insulin. Sports: bowling, cycling, skiing, swimming, tennis. "You are a person first, and your medical state should not leave you out of the mainstream of living. Pursue what you enjoy. Never hide behind your condition, but put it aside and see how you can incorporate any desires into your routine. Most of all, enjoy life."

JAMES SCHUMAN, Roxbury, New York. Age 24. Diabetic for 15 years. Treatment: insulin. Sports: skiing, biking, hiking, swimming, jogging. "You must first set your goal, the goal being that you *want* to be a well-controlled diabetic. To make this decision is a large part of the feat. Go into your sport knowing that it helps you keep yourself in control. Give your activities your best effort. Try not to get discouraged. You will soon discover the rewards of a well-balanced body."

LEONARD J. SEVERTSON, Post Falls, Idaho. Age 42. Diabetic for 10 years. Treatment: insulin. Sports: backpacking, cross-country skiing, handball. "I get satisfaction out of being able to cover more ground backpacking and cross-country skiing than most people half my age. . . . There should be no reason you can't be as active as you desire. The more the better."

DARRELL PAT SHIRES, Knoxville, Tennessee. Age 15. Diabetic for 6 years. Treatment: insulin. Sports: football, basketball, baseball, and golf. "You can compete as well as a nondiabetic with the proper care."

DAVID SILVERSTEIN, El Cerrito, California. Age 33. Diabetic for 24 years. Treatment: insulin. Sports: cycling, backpacking, folk dancing. "My sports program counterbalances the detrimental effects of eight hours a day in an office."

DAN G. SLOAN, Pittsburgh, Pennsylvania. Age 48. Diabetic for 16 years. Treatment: insulin. Sports: golf, skiing, bicycling. "Sports participation can be a real help to a newly diagnosed diabetic in overcoming the fears and uncertainties that occur when one learns he is diabetic.

Young people should be particularly encouraged to become involved in sports because it can be a real help in developing their self-confidence and in learning that diabetes does not have to limit them in enjoying a full normal life-style."

STEVEN SOUTHWICK, Baltimore, Maryland. Age 18. Diabetic for 1½ years. Treatment: insulin. Sports: skiing, bicycle racing. "Being diabetic has given me more drive in my sports to see if I can lick the handicap. It has helped me become more aware of regular exercise and diet and made me *very* regular in my exercising. This helps in any sport."

MAIDA SPERLING, Great Neck, New York. Age 38. Diabetic for 13 years. Treatment: insulin. Sports: regular physical workouts in gymnasium and tumbling. "I think that general health is vastly improved by regular exercise. All the circulatory problems are lessened when you rev up regularly. The proof of one's own possibility as an active, full-living individual is the next best lifegiving substance to insulin for a diabetic. And it's just plain fun to do."

ANITA J. SPIEGEL, Philadelphia, Pennsylvania. Age 15. Diabetic for 6 years. Treatment: insulin. Sport: ice hockey. "Diabetes doesn't interfere with anything I do. I have it and accept it. If I let it interfere with life I'd be an invalid and that would be a waste. . . . Team members I'm close with know I'm diabetic. If my being diabetic affects them then they've got a problem, not me. When I am on the ice with my team, sharing club spirit, it generates an overwhelming sensation that diabetes among other things is just stashed away in the locker room. I have two words that I urge any diabetic to try and they are *do it!*"

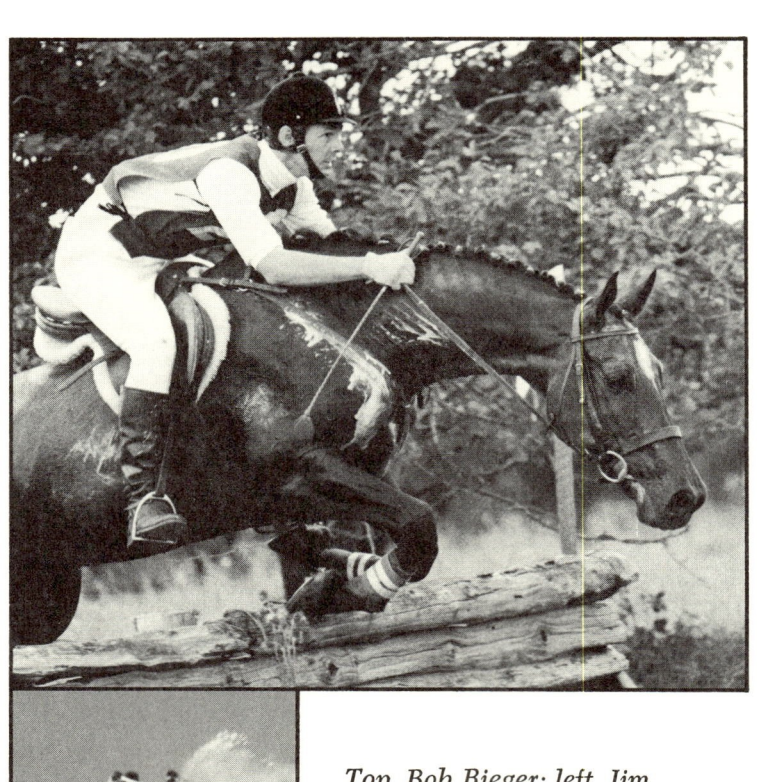

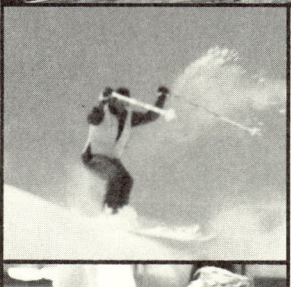

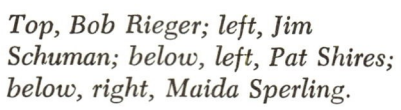

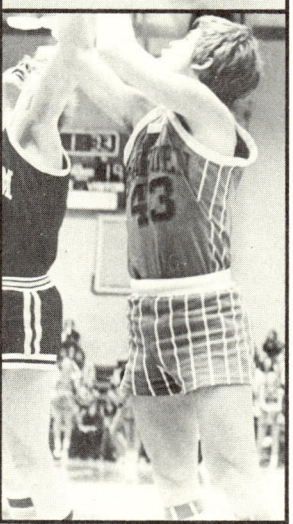

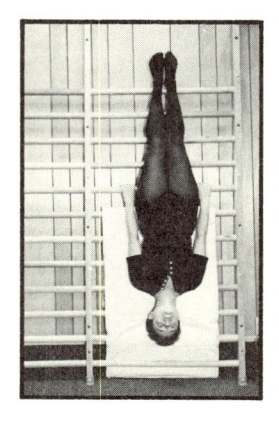

Top, Bob Rieger; left, Jim Schuman; below, left, Pat Shires; below, right, Maida Sperling.

Diabetic Doers' Profiles 233

DON L. TALBOTT, San Bernardino, California. Age 50. Diabetic for 17 years. Treatment: insulin. Sports: boating, skiing (snow and water), tennis, scuba diving. "Life is no breeze at best so do your thing the best way you can. You write your own biography and set your own goals. I've lived fifty years and enjoyed a hundred and am just starting.... I suggest that everyone must continue with certain sports and their lives will be greatly increased by their attempts."

BRENDA ("ROBIN") TALIAFERRO, Longview, Texas. Age 25. Diabetic for 17 years. Treatment: insulin. Sports: tennis, bike riding, jogging, walking, hiking, skating, bowling, exercising. "Always stay active, exercise daily, join as many sports activities as you can, follow Bill Talbert's example, and never give up!"

BRENT TAYLOR, Salt Lake City, Utah. Age 26. Diabetic for 7 years. Treatment: insulin. Sports: skiing (snow and water), hunting, fishing, basketball, football, baseball. "Start any program you feel is interesting. Begin slowly at first and be prepared. As you progress, feel or 'listen' to your body. We diabetics are, or can be, as good or better than others. We've got diets!"

JOSEPH EARL TAYLOR, JR., New Carrollton, Maryland. Age 17. Diabetic for 2½ years. Treatment: insulin. Sports: football, basketball, baseball. "Be sure you have sugar on hand while playing and try to forget about diabetes while playing. Always remember you are the same as anyone else with the exception that you have to take precautions and be a little more careful. Set your goal and work toward it. If you really are sincere in what you want to accomplish, no task will be too hard. Believe in God and have faith in your convictions. Just never give up, always give a little more than you think you can, and you'll be the best."

JEFF THOMPSON, Beulah, Michigan. Age 16. Diabetic for 2 years. Treatment: insulin. Sports: skiing, tennis, bicycling. "A diabetic can do nearly anything he wants to and should not consider himself inferior to a sports opponent if he maintains good control and eats before he exercises."

THOM UNDERWOOD, Bend, Oregon. Age 22. Diabetic for 10 years. Treatment: insulin. Sports: skiing (cross-country and downhill), rock climbing, backpacking, tennis. "Look at your advantages. Everything is still pretty together; learn what it does to you. Figure it out yourself, how your body reacts to the differences. Listen to it. It takes some time and it changes all the time. The awareness of the changes are the key. Learn these and you're unstoppable. Never use it as an excuse. If something happened wrong it's usually your fault and if you need something to save your ego besides the truth then you're backsliding. . . . Man, I got arms, legs, eyes, strong heart. Everything's there but a pancreas. Handicapped? Bah, humbug!"

MORRIS WEBER, Brooklyn, New York. Age 54. Diabetic for 15 years. Treatment: insulin. Sports: handball, paddle ball, pool, bicycling, ocean swimming. "Diabetics should participate in sports. For one thing, it is good for their blood circulation and it helps keep the diabetes under control. Also, it helps improve your mental outlook on life."

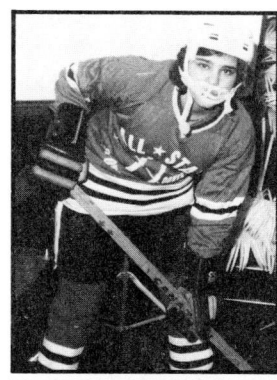

Left, Anita Spiegel; below, clockwise from left, Joe Taylor, Thom Underwood, Jean Werner.

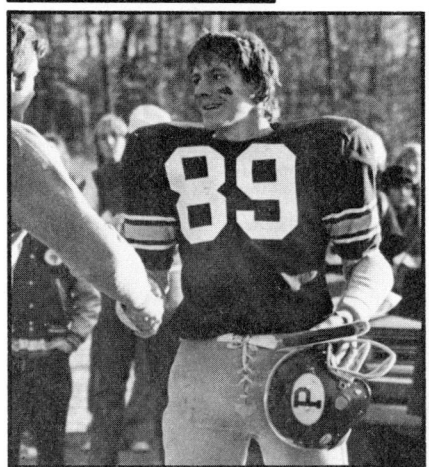

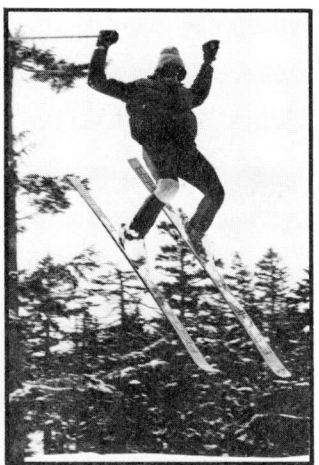

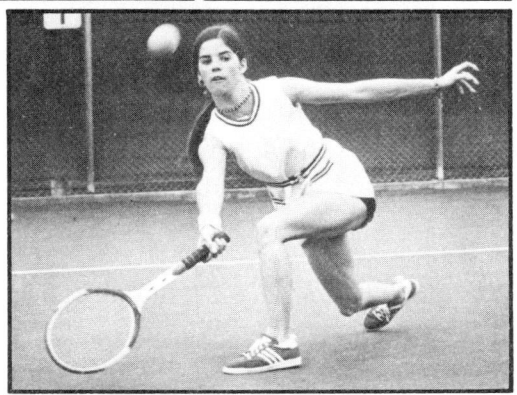

JEAN MARIE WERNER, Corona, California. Age 19. Diabetic for 10 months. Treatment: insulin. Sports: tennis, basketball. "Diabetes has made me a stronger person psychologically and probably physically also. I have learned recently from a professional player that to succeed one must set long-range goals and at the same time set short-range goals even if it is just success at each practice. These will aid tremendously in achieving that long-range goal. Diabetics may need to include goals concerning diet and conditioning, just as normal athletes. I know it can be done. My friend is the proof of what goals and determination can do."

DANIEL QUINN WICK, Spenard, Alaska. Age 15. Diabetic for 1 year. Treatment: insulin. Sports: ski racing, hunting, soccer, biking. "Don't let diabetes stop you from doing anything."

GORDON WILLE, Union Dale, Pennsylvania. Age 29. Diabetic for 13 years. Treatment: insulin. Sports: skiing, sailing, ice hockey, tennis, golf, skydiving, gliding. "Accept the fact that you're a diabetic and learn how to live a long, happy, and active life. Especially don't sit around and feel sorry for yourself. You could be a heck of a lot worse off. Don't let someone else's ignorance of diabetes deny you the chance of pursuing a particular interest. Prove to them you're capable of handling it. If you shouldn't make a team or do as well as you thought you would, practice and become better for next time. If you don't come in first, don't blame it on being diabetic. It's no excuse. Consult with a doctor and go for regular complete physicals. There is a hell of a lot to do in the world; no reason you should miss it. So take care of yourself, exercise, and enjoy."

BEVERLY WITT, Flint, Michigan. Age 35. Diabetic for 26½ years. Treatment: insulin. Sports: skiing, snowmobiling, swimming, sailing, bicycling, motorcycling. "Entering a sports or exercise program has helped very much. I feel better and I look better."

ERIKA WOLFE, Steamboat Springs, Colorado. Age 13. Diabetic for 8 years. Treatment: insulin. Sports: skiing, ice fishing, biking, swimming, hiking, baseball. "Hang in there. Even if a lot of people think you can't do it, show them you're as capable as anyone else."

Appendix **B**

Blood Pressure Chart

BLOOD PRESSURE

Age	Normal Range Systolic	Normal Range Diastolic	Age	Normal Range Systolic	Normal Range Diastolic
Men			Women		
16	105–135	60–86	16	100–130	60–85
17	105–135	60–86	17	100–130	60–85
18	105–135	60–86	18	100–130	60–85
19	105–140	60–88	19	100–130	60–85
20–24	105–140	62–88	20–24	100–130	60–85
25–29	108–140	65–90	25–29	102–130	60–86
30–34	110–145	67–92	30–34	102–135	60–88
35–39	110–145	68–92	35–39	105–140	65–90
40–44	110–150	70–94	40–44	105–150	65–92
45–49	110–155	70–96	45–49	105–155	65–96
50–54	115–160	70–98	50–54	110–165	70–100
55–59	115–165	70–98	55–59	110–170	70–100
60–64	115–170	70–100	60–64	115–175	70–100

Reprinted from the Journal of the American Medical Association, August 26, 1950, Volume 143. Copyright 1950, American Medical Association.

Appendix **C**

Cholesterol and Triglycerides

	Normal Range	
Age	Cholesterol	Triglycerides
Under 29	120–140	10–140
30–39	140–270	10–150
40–49	150–310	10–160
Over 49	160–330	10–190

Appendix D

Maximum Heartbeat

Age	Maximum Heartbeat Attainable
25	200
30	194
35	188
40	182
45	176
50	171
55	165
60	159
65	153

Appendix **E**

Chart of Calorie Expenditures

	Gross Energy Cost (Calories per Hour) [*]
Rest and Light Activity	*50–200*
Lying down or sleeping	80
Sitting	100
Driving an automobile	120
Standing	140
Domestic work	180
Moderate Activity	*200–350*
Bicycling (5½ mph)	210
Walking (2½ mph)	210
Gardening	220
Canoeing (2½ mph)	230
Golf	250
Lawn mowing (power mower)	250
Bowling	270
Lawn mowing (hand mower)	270

[*] Energy expended by a 150-pound person. The standards represent a compromise between those proposed by the British Medical Association (1950), Christensen (1953), and Wells, Balke, and Van Fossan (1956). Where available, actual measured values have been used; for other values a "best guess" was made.

	Gross Energy Cost (Calories per Hour)
Moderate Activity (cont.)	*200–350*
Fencing	300
Rowboating (2½ mph)	300
Swimming (¼ mph)	300
Walking (3¾ mph)	300
Badminton	350
Horseback riding (trotting)	350
Square dancing	350
Volleyball	350
Roller skating	350
Vigorous Activity	*over 350*
Table tennis	360
Ditch digging (hand shovel)	400
Ice skating (10 mph)	400
Wood chopping or sawing	400
Tennis	420
Waterskiing	480
Hill climbing (100 ft. per hr.)	490
Skiing (10 mph)	600
Squash and handball	600
Cycling (13 mph)	660
Scull rowing (race)	840
Running (10 mph)	900

Used with permission of R. E. Johnson.

Appendix F

Sugar Content of Various Blood-Sugar-Raising Snacks

Item	Size	Approximate Sugar Content (teaspoons)
Candy		
Hershey Bar	1⅕-oz. bar	5
Milky Way	1¹¹⁄₁₆-oz. bar	5½
Fudge	1 small piece	4½
Life Savers	1 roll	10
Candy cane	1 small	20
Sucker	1 small	5
All-day sucker	1 large	20
Marshmallow	1 piece	1½
Gumdrops	1 piece	2
Chewing gum	1 stick	½
Beverages		
Coca-Cola	12 oz.	12
Ginger ale	12 oz.	8
Sweet cider	6 oz.	5
Orangeade	6 oz.	7
Cakes, Cookies, Pies		
Angel food	1 small piece	7
Banana cake	1 small piece	4
Cheesecake	1 small piece	2
Chocolate cake	1 small piece	10
Coffee cake	1 small piece	5

Item	Size	Approximate Sugar Content (teaspoons)
Cakes, Cookies, Pies (cont.)		
Jelly roll	1 small piece	5
Cupcake	1	6
Brownie	1	4
Chocolate cookie	1	1½
Fig Newton	1	5
Gingersnap	1	3
Oatmeal cookie	1	2
Sugar cookie	1	1½
Fruit pie	⅙ medium pie	14
Raisin pie	⅙ medium pie	19
Pastries, desserts		
Chocolate eclair	1	7
Cream puff	1	2
Doughnut (plain)	1	4
Doughnut (glazed)	1	6
Doughnut (jelly)	1	7
Jell-O	½ cup	5
Chocolate pudding	½ cup	4
Ice Cream Products		
Ice cream	1 scoop	4
Sherbet	1 scoop	6
Chocolate milk	8 oz.	6
Milk shake	8 oz.	16
Jams		
Apple butter	1 tablespoon	1
Jelly, jam	1 tablespoon	4–6

Most canned fruits are packed in syrup which is high in sugar content. One cup of fruit averages from 9 to 18 teaspoons of sugar.

Courtesy of the University of Southern California School of Dentistry

Appendix **G**

What School Personnel Should Know About the Student with Diabetes

Prepared by American Diabetes Association, Committee on Diabetes in Youth; Endorsed by the National Education Association, Department of School Nurses

GENERAL INFORMATION

All school personnel (teachers, nurses, principal, lunchroom workers, playground and hall supervisors, bus drivers, counselors, etc.) *must* be informed that a student has diabetes. It is imperative all personnel understand the fundamentals of the disease and its care.

Diabetes is *NOT* an infectious disease. It results from failure of the pancreas to make a sufficient amount of insulin. Without insulin food cannot be used properly. Diabetes currently cannot be cured but can be controlled. Treatment consists of daily injections of insulin and a prescribed food plan. Children with diabetes can participate in all school activities and should not be considered different from other students. It is essential school personnel have conferences with parents early in each school year to obtain more specific information about the individual child and his specific needs. Communication and cooperation between parents and school personnel can help the diabetic child have a happy and well adjusted school experience.

INSULIN REACTIONS

Insulin reactions occur when the amount of sugar in the blood is too low. This is caused by an imbalance of insulin, too much exercise, or too little food. Under these circumstances the body sends out numerous warning signs. If these signs are recognized early, reactions may be promptly terminated by giving some form of sugar. If a reaction is not treated, unconsciousness and convulsions may result. The child may recognize many of the following warning signs of low blood sugar and should be encouraged to report them.

WARNING SIGNS OF INSULIN REACTIONS

Excessive Hunger	Blurred Vision	Poor Coordination
Perspiration	Irritability	Abdominal Pain
Pallor	Crying	or Nausea
Headache	Confusion	Inappropriate
Dizziness	Inability to	Actions/Responses
Nervousness or Trembling	Concentrate	
	Drowsiness or Fatigue	

TREATMENT

At the first sign of any of the above warning signs:
  Give sugar immediately in one of the following forms:
  a. Sugar—5 small cubes, 2 packets, or 2 teaspoons
  b. Fruit juice—½ to ⅔ cup
  c. Carbonated beverage *(not diet or sugarless soda pop)*—6 ounces
  d. Candy—¼ to ⅓ candy bar

The student experiencing a reaction may need coaxing to eat. If improvement does not occur within 15-20 minutes, repeat the feeding. If the child does not improve after administration of the second feeding containing sugar, the parents or physician should be called. When the child improves, he should be given a small feeding of ½ sandwich and a glass of milk. He should then resume normal school activities and the parents advised of the incident.

DIET

Children with diabetes follow a prescribed diet and may select their foods from the school lunch menu or bring their own lunch. Lunchroom managers should be made aware of the child's dietary needs, which may include midmorning and midafternoon snacks to help avoid insulin reactions. Adequate time should be provided for finishing meals.

URINE TESTING

The amount of sugar in the urine of a child with diabetes reflects the level of sugar in the blood. Testing the urine for sugar several times a day serves as an effective guide to proper diabetes control. Urine tests for sugar should be made before meals, and time should be allowed before lunch for the diabetic child to perform this test if requested.

GENERAL ADVICE

The child with diabetes should be carefully observed in class, particularly before lunch. It is best not to schedule physical education just before lunch; and if possible the child should not be assigned to a late lunch period. Many children require nourishment before strenuous exercise. Teachers and nurses should have sugar available at all times. The child with diabetes should also carry a sugar supply and be permitted to treat a reaction when it occurs.

Diabetic coma, a serious complication of the disease, results from uncontrolled diabetes. This does *NOT* come on suddenly and generally need not be a concern to school personnel.

The following information should be obtained from parents when conference is held at the beginning of the school term.

Child's Name		Date	
Parent's Name		Address	Phone
Alternate person to call in emergency		Relationship	Phone
Physician's Name		Address	Phone

Signs and symptoms the child usually exhibits preceding insulin reaction:_____

Time of day reaction most likely to occur:_____
Most effective treatment (sweets most readily accepted):

Kind of morning or afternoon snack: _____

Suggested "treats" for in-school parties: _____

Substitute and/or special teachers should have access to the above information.

This material may be reprinted for the child's cumulative school record. For additional information or copies of this card, contact: American Diabetes Association, 1 West 48th Street, New York, New York 10020

Courtesy of the American Diabetes Association

Index

Italic page numbers indicate illustrations

ADA *Forecast*, 51
Adams, Clara, 205
Adidas sports shoes, 119
Adrenaline, 74, 75
Airplane, diabetics restricted from flying, 180–81
Alarie, Thomas Joseph, 205
Albert, June, 123–26, 205–6, *210*
Albright, Tenley, M.D., 142, 195
Alexander, Ralph, M.D., 38
American Diabetes Association (ADA), 17, 68, 135, 152, 153, 173
American Podiatry Association, 120
Ames Company, 86, 87, 88
Anderson, Tim W., 206
Archery, 207, 212
Arteriosclerosis, 43
Arthritis, 129
Atherosclerosis, 44
Athlete's foot, 120–21, 163
Austin, Betsy, 206, *210*

Backpacking, 184, 187, 206, 211, 212, 217, 221, 228, 230, 234; diabetic supplies for, 102
Badminton, 206, 214, 227
Baseball, 13, 60, 72, 73, 92, 171, 182, 205, 206, 208, 211, 217, 222, 224, 230, 233, 237; Little League, 157
Basketball, 205, 207, 209, 211, 214, 216, 218, 222, 225, 227, 230, 233, 236
Beamsderfer, Virginia Maggio, 207
Bernstein, Dick, 35, 42, 43, 46, 54, 58, 88, 89, 96 *97*, 98, 134, 140, 141, 142, 189, 191, 192, 193, 207; quoted, 44–45
"Bernstein" exercises, 140–42
Bicycle racing, 231
Bicycling, 134, 135–36, 187, 205–6, 208, 209, 213, 214, 216, 217, 221, 223, 224, 228, 229, 230, 233, 234, 236, 237
Bisesti, Paul T., 207
Black, Janet, 207
Blackburn, Mark A., 207–8
Blindness, 49
Blood pressure chart, 238
Blood sugar, measurement of, 86–88
Boating, 207, 233
Bowling, 207, 212, 224, 225, 228, 229, 233
Brink, Joe ("Mr. Cincinnati"), 34, 39, 54, 58, 67, 68, 96, 182, 191, 192, *193*, 208, *210*
Brutsche, Joan Linn, 208
Buerger-Allen exercises, 139–40, 142

Caine, Lynn, quoted, 51

250

Index

Calisthenics, 133, 143; *see also* Exercise(s)
Calorie expenditures, chart of, 241–42
Campbell, Laila M., 111, 112, 208, *210*
Camping, 207, 212, 214, 222, 228
Camps for diabetic children, 153–56
Canfield & Company, C. R., 79
Canoeing, 208, 212, 217, 225
Carbohydrates, as source of energy, 115
Carey, Dave, 208–9
Carruthers, Malcolm, M.D., 50
Cass, John E., 209
Chocolate candy, for raising blood sugar, 82
Cholesterol, 44, 45, 46, 239
Clark, Brent, 209, *210*
Clarke, Bobby, 13, 22, 63, 113, 172, 174, *183*, 184
Coaches, sports, and diabetics, 170–78
Colonel Sanders, 79–80
Colorimeter, 88
Coma, diabetic, 49, 86, 248; *see also* Hyperglycemia
Conley, Gail Dietz, 209
Cooper, Jerry M., 209, 211
Creighton, Norma, 211
CRIPE program(s), 130–37, 142; different activities for, 133–38
Crowling, Robert Keith, 211
Cutter, Gregory, 211

D.B.I., 37, 123
Deaconess Hospital (Spokane), 32, 79, 83
Decubitus ulcers, 139, 140
Devine, Anna, 212
Dextrose cubes, for raising blood sugar, 79
Dextrostix, 85, 86, 87, 88
Diabetes: advantages of having, 192–201; complications of, 43, 49, 148; disadvantages of having, 180–92; as healthiest disease, 195–97; and interference with sports, 185–92; juvenile-onset, *see* Juvenile-onset diabetes; maturity-onset, 36, 38, 46, 48, 50, 55, 122, 142; self-discipline taught by, 193–95; specialists for treating, 167, 168; and stress, 50; students with, and information for school personnel, 245–49; telling others about, 90–95
Diabetes Association of Greater Cleveland, 78
Diabetes Education Center (Deaconess Hospital), 32, 83
Diabetes Forecast, 22, 36, 86, 154
Diabetes in the News, 22
Diabetes Question and Answer Book, The (Biermann and Toohey), 23, 173
Diabetes Teaching Guide (Joslin Clinic), 83
Diabetic Care in Pictures (Helen and Joseph Rosenthal), 188
Directory of Medical Specialists, 168
Doctors, 158–70
Driscoll, Richard Charles, 212, *215*

Endurance training, 131
Engerbretson, David L., 14, 31, 32, 33, 34, 39, 40, 84, 98, 102, 103–4, 105, 118, 129, 130, 132, 133, 162, 174, 175, 176, 184, 199, 212
Epley, Dick, 212–13
Estes, Elaine, 213
Exercise(s): Bernstein's, 140–42; Buerger-Allen, 139–40, 142; and companionship, 95–99; continuous, 130–31; and diet, normal, 49; for elderly, 129, 132, 133, 136, 138–41; and emergency rations, 109; and endurance, 131; and food intake, increase of, 62–64; and heart attack, reducing risk of, 44; in intervals, 131, 132; insulin reactions as result of, 31, 32–33, 36, 59, 61–62; as "invisible insulin," 33–34, 41; after meal, as safest time, 107–8;

Exercise(s) (cont.)
  mental-health values of, 51;
  norepinephrine released by, 50; and oral hypoglycemic agents, 37–38; progressive, 131, 133; rhythmical, 131; snacks while doing, see Snacks for diabetics; spilling prevented by, 41; and weight problems, 38–40, 46, 47, 48; see also Calisthenics; CRIPE program(s); Insulin reactions; Sports

Farrell, Maureen, R.N., quoted, 154–55
Fats, as source of energy, 115
Fear, reactions to, 74–76
Federal Aviation Agency (FAA), 181, 182
Feet, care of, 119
Fencing, 225
Field hockey, 206, 207, 214, 223
Fishing, 212, 216–17, 221, 222, 227, 229, 233, 237
Fitness, physical, how to get, 129–45
Flying (power and glider), 181, 211
Folk dancing, 230
Food and Drug Administration (FDA), 37
Food Exchange System, 17
Football, 65, 161, 176, 177, 191, 205, 206, 208, 211, 217, 225, 230, 233
Frank, Dorothy, 213
Fredericks, Carlton, quoted, 166–67
Fruit juices, for raising blood sugar, 80
Fulvicin, 121

Gangrene, 49, 121, 148, 188
Gardening, 228
Gatorade, 82
Gerner, Lee, 213, *215*
Glucagon, 76–77, 111, 175, 176
Gluconeogenesis, 115

Glucose, 41, 57, 75, 76; in blood, 33, 36, 48, 57, 75; instant, 78
Glycogen, 41, 42
Glycogenolysis, 41
Godfrey, Lisa, 213–14
Golf, 186, 200, 209, 211, 212, 213, 217, 218, 221, 222, 223, 227, 228, 229, 230, 236
Goodhart, Marcia, 214, *215*
Goos, Rolf A., 214, *215*
Gornell, John, 214
Grape juice, for raising blood sugar, 80
Gwinup, Grant, M.D., 50

Hage, Sandra Fay, 214, 216, *219*
Halftime Punch, 82
Handball, 161, 211, 218, 228, 230, 234
Hangnails, 188
Harris, Theresa, 73, 178, 216, *219*; quoted, 178–79
Havlicak, Vince E., 216, *219*
Hayes, Karen, 216
Head, Eric, 216–17
Healing of diabetic's injuries, 188–91
Heart attack, 44
Heart rate, 140, 141; maximum, 240
Hicks, Mike, 217
High blood pressure, 44
Hiking, 207, 208, 211, 214, 221, 222, 223, 225, 228, 229, 230, 233, 237
Hilts, Eric Wade, 217
Hockey, 13, 63, 113, 161, 176, 182, 184, 201, 231, 236
Honey, for raising blood sugar, 79–80, 83
Hopkins, Jacqueline, 217
Horse training, 218, 227
Horseback riding, 214, 221, 225, 227
Humphreys, Dick, 217–18, *219*
Hunting, 212, 216, 223, 229, 233, 236
Hyperglycemia, 74, 86, 190; see also Coma, diabetic
Hypertension, 44

Index

Hypoglycemia, 57, 58, 59, 61, 74, 82, 86, 87, 115; *see also* Insulin reactions; Shock, insulin
Hypoglycemic agents, oral, 37, 38

Ice fishing, 237
Ice skating, 206, 214, 224
Identification, diabetic, 100–101
Infection, 58, 165, 169, 188, 190, 191
Instant glucose, 78
Insulin: increasing costliness of, 34; "invisible," exercise as, 33–34, 41; Lente, 68; no need to keep cool, 117–19; NPH, 32, 68, 153; reductions of, as result of exercise, 31, 32–33, 36, 59, 61–62
Insulin reactions, 34, 41, 42, 57–59, 60, 61, 67, 68–71, 84, 92, 109, 112, 148, 159, 246, 247; overkilling, 84–85; during summertime, 71–74; treatment of, 246; warning signs of, 246; *see also* Hypoglycemia; Shock, insulin
Isometrics, 213

Jam and jelly, for raising blood sugar, 83
Jogging, 97, 132, 133, 134, 136, 206, 207, 212, 213, 217, 223, 225, 228, 230, 233
Johnson, Perry, quoted, 108
Johnson, Richard, 218
Joslin, Elliott, M.D., 122
Joslin Clinic, 83, 137
Journal of the American Medical Association, 134
Journey, 194
Jumping rope, 134–35, 208
Juvenile Diabetes Foundation, 152
Juvenile-onset diabetes, 36, 38, 45, 122, 191; and camps for children, 153–56; diet for, at school, 247; information on, for school personnel, 245–49; insulin reactions in, 246; and mothers' attitudes, *see* Mothers of diabetic children; urine testing in, 247

Kadwit, Betsy, 218
Kalkin, Alan S., 218, *226*
Karate, 211, 218, 227
Karo syrup, for raising blood sugar, 82, 83
Kayaking, 217
Ketones, 153, 165
Ketostix, 87
Kidney disease, 49
Kite flying, 227
Krall, Leo, M.D., 36
Krueger, Joyce V., 218, 220

Lactic acid cycle, 42
Larson, Roger C., 59, 60, 139, 140
Lawlor, Marnie, 220
Lawn bowling, 205
Lawrence, Ronald A., M.D., 128
Leete, Edward, 43, 45–46, 49, 50, 63, 107, 108, 220
Lente insulin, 68
Lewis, Frank, 174
Life Savers, for raising blood sugar, 81–82, 83, 84, 151, 164
Linderholm, Muriel, 220
Lomen, Lynn, 110
Low Blood Sugar Emergencies in the Diabetic Child (film), 152, 174
Lowenkopf, Shelly, 23, 126–29, 163, 221
Lurie, Stephen Jon, 221

McDonald's restaurants, 135
McGurrin, Thomas M., 221
McNally, Mike, 221–22
McNutt, Mike, 222
Markovich, Tom, Jr., 222
Martin, Mike, 222–23
Maslow, Abraham, 217
Massie, Bobby, 194
Matson, Glenn A., 223
Maturity-onset diabetes, 36, 38, 46, 48, 50, 55, 122, 142
Maxwell, John, 223
Mayer, Jean, 46, 47, 48
Medic Alert (Foundation), 100–101, 110
Melnyk, Gerry, 184
Menses, Carol, 223

Mirsky, Stanley, 86
Moll, Patricia, 223–24, *226*
Money, importance of carrying by diabetic, 101–2
Moore, Mary Tyler, 143, *144*, 196
Morehouse, Lawrence, 108
Morris, Brian, 224
Mothers of diabetic children, 147–58; information supplied by, 151–52; positive approach by, 148–49, 151; and summer camps, 153–56
Motorcycling, 211, 216, 228, 237
Mountain climbing, 159, 160, 206, 225
Muscle mass, in diabetic, 191–92

Naruk, Stephen, 13, 14, 224, *226*
Needlepoint, Camp, 154
Nelson, Brian Anthony, 224–25
New York Diabetes Association, 154
Norepinephrine, 50
Nottingham, Cynthia, 225
NPH insulin, 32, 68, 153
Nutrition Handbook, The (Fredericks), 166

O'Brien, Coley, 149, *150*
Olson, O. Charles, M.D., 32, 57, 74, 79, 82, 83, 115, 134, 189, 190, 192
Oral hypoglycemic agents, 37, 38
Orange juice, for raising blood sugar, 80, 83, 85, 151
Orinase, 33, 34, 37, 123
Osgood, Patricia, 225, *226*

Pancreas, hormones from, 77
Parachute jumping, 181
Pedometer, 138
Pills (oral hypoglycemic agents), 37, 38
Pilot, aircraft, diabetic, 181
Pine, Susan, 225
Ping-Pong, 217
Pirman, Helen, 227
Platform tennis, 214
Playing for Life (Talbert), 22
Podiatry, 119–20

Pool, 234
Poucher, Russell, M.D., 68, 69, 80, 121
Principles of Modern Physical Education, Health, and Recreation (Updyke and Johnson), 108
Proteins, and gluconeogenesis, 115

Quinn, Becki, 227

Reactose, 79
Reeder, Kenneth R., 227
Respiratory problem, during shock, 111–12
Retinal hemorrhage, 140
Rhodes, Lewis A., 152
Rieger, Bob, 227, *232*
Robinson, Jackie, 184
Robles, Frank H., 227–28
Rock climbing, 224, 234
Rodeo riding, 216
Rollerskating, 214
Rope jumping, 134–35, 208
Rosenberg, Jo, 228
Rosenthal, Helen, 188
Rosenthal, Joseph, M.D., 188
Rowan, Dan, 32, 62, 143, *145*
Rowing, 207
Rowley, Durwood B., 228
Royal Canadian Air Force Exercise Plans for Physical Fitness, 40, 133
Ruderman, Neil, M.D., quoted, 36
Rugby, 224
Running, 97, 133, 194–95, 196, 207, 209, 214, 218, 220, 221, 225
Ryan, R. J., 228–29

Sailing, 206, 207, 211, 222, 224, 236, 237
Santo, Ron, 13, 22, 56, 60, 72, 73, 92, 94, 199
Schlappal, Deborah Lynn, 229
Schmetter, Dean, 229
Scholer, Arlene Margaret, 229
School personnel, information for, on students with diabetes, 245–49

Index

Schuman, James, 230, 232
Scuba diving, 178–79, 209, 211, 216, 233
Severtson, Leonard J., 230
Shires, Darrell Pat, 230, 232
Shock, insulin, 34, 41, 57, 58, 69, 71, 74, 75, 77, 86, 92, 109, 110, 111, 151; see also Hypoglycemia; Insulin reactions
Shoes for diabetics, 119
Silverstein, David, 230
Sims, Ethan, M.D., quoted, 51
Ski racing, 236
Skiing, 141, 160, 161, 194, 200, 206, 207, 208, 209, 211, 212, 213, 214, 216, 217, 218, 220, 221, 222, 223, 224, 225, 227, 228, 229, 230, 231, 233, 234, 236, 237; and emergency rations, 109; on Gibson Pass, 111–12
Skydiving, 181, 182, 236
Sloan, Dan G., 230–31
Snacks for diabetics, 112–15; list of, 114; sugar content of, 243–44
Snowmobiling, 237
Snowshoeing, 222
Soccer, 236
Soft drinks, for raising blood sugar, 80–81, 83, 151
Softball, 214, 223, 225
Southwick, Steven, 231
Specialists for diabetes, 167, 168
Spelunking, 212
Sperling, Maida, 231, 232
Spiegel, Anita J., 231, 235
Spilling, 35, 41, 59, 65, 66, 85, 86, 123; taste test for, 89
Sportade, 82
Sports: calorie expenditures for, 241–42; coaches in, and diabetics, 170–78; companionship in, 95–99; diabetes' interference with, 185–92; diabetic supplies for, overpreparation of, 103–5; list of, 52–53; snacks during, see Snacks for diabetics; see also Exercise(s); Insulin reactions

Sports friends for diabetics, 54–56, 90–94, 116–17
Sportscar driving, 212
Squash, 227
Stiles, Merritt, M.D., 160
Stress, and diabetes, 50
Sugar: in blood, see Glucose, in blood; to counteract insulin reactions, 81, 83, 84, 85
Sugar content, in snacks for diabetics, 243–44
Surfing, 211
Swimming, 134, 170, 171, 196, 206, 207, 208, 211, 214, 216, 217, 218, 221, 222, 223, 224, 225, 228, 229, 230, 234, 237; after meals, 108
Syrup, maple, for raising blood sugar, 83

Talbert, Bill, 20, 22, 24, 25, 63, 65, 137, 147, 193, 197, 233
Talbott, Don L., 233
Taliaferro, Brenda ("Robin"), 233
Taste test for spilling, 89
Taylor, Brent, 233
Taylor, Joseph Earl, Jr., 233–34, 235
Tennis, 20, 22, 147, 186, 187, 188, 197, 205, 206, 207, 208, 211, 213, 214, 217, 218, 220, 221, 222, 224, 228, 229, 233, 234, 236
Tes-Tape, 18, 19, 20, 65, 88
Thompson, Jeff, 234
Thrombophlebitis, 140
Tiger sports shoes, 119
Tinactin, 121
Tobogganing, 214, 217
Track events, 209, 213, 214, 218, 225
Tretorn sports shoes, 119
Triglycerides, 44, 45, 46, 239
Tumbling, 231

Ulcers, decubitus, 139, 140
Underwood, Thom, 78, 81, 91, 119, 164, 184, 196, 198, 234, 235
Updyke, Wynn, quoted, 108

Urine test, 85, 86, 88–89, 247; and "second void," 86

Van Dellen, Theodore, 156
Volleyball, 206, 214, 225, 227

Walking, 134, 136–38, 213, 220, 223, 227, 228, 233
Water skiing, 213, 216, 218, 223, 227, 233
Weber, Morris, 234
Weight lifting, 34, 54, 96, 191, 192, 207, 208, 213, 216
Weight Lifting Machine, Universal, 97
Weight problems, and exercise, 38–40, 46, 47, 48
Werner, Jean Marie, 235, 236
Whitaker, Camp, 154
Wick, Daniel Quinn, 236
Widow (Caine), 51
Wille, Gordon, 236–37
Witt, Beverly, 237
Wolfe, Erika, 237
Wrestling, 65, 161, 176, 186, 217

Zohman, Lenore, M.D., 44